NEW APPROACHES IN CANCER THERAPY

*Monograph Series of the European
Organization for Research on Treatment of Cancer
Volume 11*

MONOGRAPH SERIES OF THE EUROPEAN ORGANIZATION FOR RESEARCH ON TREATMENT OF CANCER

The Monograph Series of the EORTC deals with selected topics related to cancer treatment. Volumes are usually, but not necessarily, based on the proceedings of an EORTC symposium. The responsibility of the Editorial Advisory Board is to approve the subject of each monograph; the Board does not review individual manuscripts.

New Approaches in Cancer Therapy

Monograph Series of the European Organization for Research on Treatment of Cancer
Volume 11

Editors

H. Cortés Funes, M. D., Ph.D.
Sección Oncología Médica
Hospital "1º de Octubre"
Universidad Complutense
Madrid, Spain

M. Rozencweig, M. D.
Department of Chemotherapy
Institut Jules Bordet
Tumor Center of the Free
University of Brussels
Brussels, Belgium

Raven Press ■ New York

Raven Press, 1140 Avenue of the Americas, New York, New York 10036

Great care has been taken to maintain the accuracy of the information contained in the volume. However, Raven Press cannot be held responsible for errors or for any consequences arising from the use of the information contained herein.

Library of Congress Cataloging in Publication Data
Main entry under title:

New approaches in cancer therapy.

(Monograph series of the European Organization for Research on Treatment of Cancer ; v. 11)
    Includes index.
    1. Cancer—Chemotherapy.   2. Antineoplastic agents—Testing.   3. Chemotherapy, Combination—Evaluation.
I. Funes, H. Cortés.   II. Rozencweig, M. (Marcel)
III. Series.   [DNLM: 1. Neoplasms—Drug therapy—Congresses.   2. Anti-neoplastic agents—Congresses.   3. Clinical trials—Congresses.   W1 N0559U v.11 / QZ 267 N5315 1980]
RC271.C5N45   616.99'4061   81-40201
ISBN 0-89004-781-2

Preface

Recent advances in cancer chemotherapy have generated new hopes for cure in patients with malignant diseases. Progress has been obtained through the identification of new active agents, better understanding of their mechanisms of action, and clearer elucidation of drug disposition and metabolism. Increasingly effective combination chemotherapy regimens and their incorporation into combined modality approaches have further expanded the grounds for therapeutic success.

This volume, based on a symposium recently organized by the European Organization for Research on Treatment of Cancer in Madrid, Spain, emphasizes new agents that have shown a significant impact in cancer chemotherapy. Authoritative chapters cover the latest advances in drug therapy for a variety of tumor types and combined modality strategies against solid malignancies. These chapters provide insight into research trends and the ingredients for their successful application, and should prove of great interest to oncologists and general internists.

Cancer therapy is a rapidly evolving area of research. We hope that the reader will recognize the foundations of the future in light of the new orientations for therapeutic modalities that are indicated in this volume.

H. Cortés Funes, M.D., Ph.D.
M. Rozencweig, M.D.

Contents

Contributors

Reto Abele
Division of Oncology
University Hospital
Ch-1211 Geneva 4 Switzerland

Pierre Alberto
Division of Oncology
University Hospital
Ch-1211 Geneva 4 Switzerland

R. J. Aur
St. Jude Children's Research Hospital
332 North Lauderdale, P. O. Box 318
Memphis, Tennessee 38101

Thomas L. Avery
St. Jude Children's Research Hospital
332 North Lauderdale, P. O. Box 318
Memphis, Tennessee 38101

G. Bonadonna
Istituto Nazionale Tumori
Via Venezian, 1
20133 Milan, Italy

Joseph Bottino
Division of Oncology
Department of Medicine
New York University Medical Center
New York, New York 10016

W. P. Bowman
St. Jude Children's Research Hospital
332 North Lauderdale, P. O. Box 318
Memphis, Tennessee 38101

C. Brambilla
Istituto Nazionale Tumori
Via Venezian, 1
20133 Milan, Italy

V. H. C. Bramwell
Cancer Research Campaign
Department of Medical Oncology
Manchester University, Christie Hospital,
*   and Holt Radium Institute*
Manchester, United Kingdom

K. Brunner
Division of Oncology
Inselspital
Bern, Switzerland

U. Bruntsch
5, Medizinische Klinik
Nurnberg, West Germany

Fernando Camacho
Department of Oncology
Montefiore Hospital and Medical Center
Gun Hill Road
Bronx, New York 10467

Antonio Canalog
Department of Gynecology
Albert Einstein College of Medicine
1300 Morris Park Avenue
Bronx, New York 10461

E. S. Casper
Developmental Chemotherapy
Solid Tumor and Clinical Immunology
*   Services*
Department of Medicine
Memorial Sloan-Kettering Cancer Center
Cornell University Medical College
New York, New York 10021

Franco Cavalli
Division of Oncology
Ospedale San Giovanni
6500 Bellinzona, Switzerland

R. A. Chapman
Developmental Chemotherapy
Solid Tumor and Clinical Immunology
  Services
Department of Medicine
Memorial Sloan-Kettering Cancer Center
Cornell University Medical College
New York, New York 10021

M. Clavel
Centre Léon Bérard
Lyon, France

H. Cortés Funes
Sección de Oncología Médica
Ciudad Sanitaria de la Seguridad Social
  "1° de Octubre"
Carretera de Andalucia Km 5.5
Madrid 17, Spain

Gary V. Dahl
St. Jude Children's Research Hospital
332 North Lauderdale, P. O. Box 318
Memphis, Tennessee 38101

O. Dalesio
EORTC/Data Center
Brussels, Belgium

Pierre Dodion
University of Maryland Cancer Center
22 South Green Street
Baltimore, Maryland 21201

Lawrence H. Einhorn
Department of Medicine
Indiana University Medical Center, and
Indianapolis Veteran's Administration
  Medical Center
Indianapolis, Indiana 46223

J. Estapé
Sección de Coodinación Oncológica
Hospital Clínico y Provincial
Barcelona, Spain

M. Fernandez Vega
Hospital Oncológico Provincial
C/Maiquez, 7
Madrid 9, Spain

W. Gallmeier
5, Medizinische Klinik
Nurnberg, West Germany

B. Gignoux
Centre Léon Bérard
Lyon, France

R. B. Golbey
Developmental Chemotherapy
Solid Tumor and Clinical Immunology
  Services
Department of Medicine
Memorial Sloan-Kettering Cancer Center
Cornell University Medical College
New York, New York 10021

R. J. Gralla
Developmental Chemotherapy
Solid Tumor and Clinical Immunology
  Services
Department of Medicine
Memorial Sloan-Kettering Cancer Center
Cornell University Medical College
New York, New York 10021

Edward Greenwald
Department of Medicine
Albert Einstein College of Medicine
1300 Morris Park Avenue
Bronx, New York 10461

L. M. Itri
Developmental Chemotherapy
Solid Tumor and Clinical Immunology
  Services
Department of Medicine
Memorial Sloan-Kettering Cancer Center
Cornell University Medical College
New York, New York 10021

F. Jungi
Division of Oncology
Kantonsspital
St. Gallen, Switzerland

Barry H. Kaplan
Department of Medicine
Albert Einstein College of Medicine
1300 Morris Park Avenue
Bronx, New York 10461

D. P. Kelsen
Developmental Chemotherapy
Solid Tumor and Clinical Immunology
  Services
Department of Medicine
Memorial Sloan-Kettering Cancer Center
Cornell University Medical College
New York, New York 10021

Yvon Kenis
Department of Chemotherapy
Institut Jules Bordet
Centre des Tumeurs de l'Université
  Libre de Bruxelles
Laboratoire d'Investigation Clinique
  H. J. Tagnon
Rue Héger-Bordet
Brussels, Belgium

A. Kirkpatrick
EORTC/Data Center
Brussels, Belgium

S. E. Krown
Developmental Chemotherapy
Solid Tumor and Clinical Immunology
  Services
Department of Medicine
Memorial Sloan-Kettering Cancer Center
Cornell University Medical College
New York, New York 10021

J. Lankelma
The Netherlands Cancer Institute
Plesmanlaan 121
1066 CX Amsterdam, The Netherlands

O. Leiva
Hospital "1° de Octubre"
Carretera de Andalucia Km 5.5
Madrid, Spain

A. Leyva
The Netherlands Cancer Institute
Plesmanlaan 121
1066 CX Amsterdam, The Netherlands

A. Thomas Look
St. Jude Children's Research Hospital
332 North Lauderdale, P. O. Box 318
Memphis, Tennessee 38101

G. R. Lynch
Developmental Chemotherapy
Solid Tumor and Clinical Immunology
  Services
Department of Medicine
Memorial Sloan-Kettering Cancer Center
Cornell University Medical College
New York, New York 10021

P. Madrigal Alonso
Hospital Oncológico Provincial
C/Maiquez, 7
Madrid 9, Spain

S. Marchini
Istituto Nazionale Tumori
Via Venezian, 1
20133 Milan, Italy

G. Martz
Division of Oncology
Kantonsspital
Zürich, Switzerland

J. G. McVie
The Netherlands Cancer Institute
Plesmanlaan 121
1066 CX Amsterdam, The Netherlands

M. Mendez
Hospital "1° de Octubre"
Carretera de Andalucia Km 5.5
Madrid, Spain

C. Mendiola
Hospital "1° de Octubre"
Carretera de Andalucia Km 5.5
Madrid, Spain

A. Millá
Sección de Coordinacción Oncológica
Hospital Clínico y Provincial
Barcelona, Spain

Mamdouh Moukhtar
Department of Gynecology
Albert Einstein College of Medicine
1300 Morris Park Avenue
Bronx, New York 10461

A. Moyano
Baltimore Cancer Research Program
22 South Green Street
University of Maryland
Baltimore, Maryland 21201

Franco M. Muggia
Division of Oncology
Department of Medicine
New York University Medical Center
New York, New York 10016

Sharon B. Murphy
St. Jude Children's Research Hospital
332 North Lauderdale, P.O. Box 318
Memphis, Tennessee 38101

Claude Nicaise
Department of Chemotherapy
Institut Jules Bordet
Centre des Tumeurs de l'Université
  Libre de Bruxelles
Laboratoire d'Investigation Clinique
  H.J. Tagnon
Rue Héger-Bordet
Brussels, Belgium

G. Perez Manga
Hospital Oncológico Provincial
C/Maiquez, 7
Madrid 9, Spain

Martine Piccart
Department of Chemotherapy
Centre des Tumeurs de l'Université
  Libre de Bruxelles
Laboratoire d'Investigation Clinique
  H.J. Tagnon
Rue Héger-Bordet
Brussels, Belgium

H.M. Pinedo
The Netherlands Cancer Institute
Plesmanlaan 121
1066 CX Amsterdam, The Netherlands

Charles B. Pratt
St. Jude Children's Research Hospital
332 North Lauderdale, P.O. Box 318
Memphis, Tennessee 38101

Gaston Rivera
St. Jude Children's Research Hospital
332 North Lauderdale, P.O. Box 318
Memphis, Tennessee 38101

A. Rossi
Istituto Nazionale Tumori
Via Venezian, 1
20133 Milan, Italy

Marcel Rozencweig
Department of Chemotherapy
Institut Jules Bordet
Centre des Tumeurs de l'Université
  Libre de Bruxelles
Laboratoire d'Investigation Clinique
  H.J. Tagnon
Rue Héger-Bordet
Brussels, Belgium

J.M. Segovia Arana
Department of Medicine
Universidad Autónoma
Madrid, Spain

Vicki Seltzer
Department of Gynecology
Albert Einstein College of Medicine
1300 Morris Park Avenue
Bronx, New York 10461

Hans Jörg Senn
Division of Oncology
Kantonsspital
9006 St. Gallen, Switzerland

J.V. Simone
St. Jude Children's Research Hospital
332 North Lauderdale, P.O. Box 318
Memphis, Tennessee 38101

Roland W. Sonntag
Division of Oncology
University Clinics
Inselspital
3010 Bern, Switzerland

James L. Speyer
Division of Oncology
Department of Medicine
New York University Medical Center
New York, New York 10016

M. B. Stoopler
Developmental Chemotherapy
Solid Tumor and Clinical Immunology
  Services
Department of Medicine
Memorial Sloan-Kettering Cancer Center
Cornell University Medical College
New York, New York 10021

G. Stoter
The Netherlands Cancer Institute
Plesmanlaan 121
1066 CX Amsterdam, The Netherlands

G. Tancini
Istituto Nazionale Tumori
Via Venezian, 1
20133 Milan, Italy

W. W. ten Bokkel Huinink
The Netherlands Cancer Institute
Plesmanlaan 121
1066 CX Amsterdam, The Netherlands

P. Valagussa
Istituto Nazionale Tumori
Via Venezian, 1
20133 Milan, Italy

Steven E. Vogl
Department of Medicine
Albert Einstein College of Medicine
1300 Morris Park Avenue
Bronx, New York 10461

J. Wildiers
Akademisch Ziekenhuis St Rafael
Leuven, Belgium

Stephen D. Williams
Department of Medicine
Indiana University Medical Center and
Indianapolis Veteran's Administration
  Medical Center
Indianapolis, Indiana 46223

Introduction

As clinical trials in cancer chemotherapy have become increasingly complicated and precise, great effort has been devoted to the exchange of information on research methods and means. This emphasis on collaboration, first put to use in oncology and now making inroads into other medical fields, is being realized through inter-departmental, interinstitutional, and international programs. The impact of these programs on improved patient care and on scientific progress has been great. Of particular importance has been the effect on clinical trials, which require strong analytical methods identifying significant data and relationships and which cannot be carried out, or are at least very difficult to verify, without solid statistical support.

The European Organization for Research and Treatment of Cancer (EORTC) was founded in 1962 for the purpose of managing, developing, and stimulating European research activities in the clinical and experimental areas of cancer treatment. The symposium on which this volume is based was sponsored by the EORTC. Discussions and exchange of ideas and experience during this symposium were extremely useful, particularly for the young specialists in the field of medical oncology.

MEDICAL ONCOLOGY IN SPAIN

In Spain, as in other countries, medical oncology is a recently developed medical field which is still growing and expanding, although with some difficulty due to problems in precisely defining its role and its areas of application. Great expansion has occurred in all patient care facilities during the last 15 years, and the new Spanish hospital system has made possible adequate teaching in all areas of medicine and surgery involving multidisciplinary postgraduate training programs. The development of internal medicine, hematology, radiology, surgery, and, in some hospitals, immunology services has produced greater interest in the diagnosis and treatment of tumors. This interest has led to the formation of separate oncology services and to the organization of cooperative groups of specialists from a variety of fields.

These developments seem very promising when considering the current status and the probable evolution of medical oncology in Spain. However, they would be far from sufficient without a clear understanding among all interested parties of the essential need to collaborate with particular respect to program planning and execution. Common protocols have already been initiated in several hospitals, but this is only a first step which must be followed by many more. In this regard, the EORTC Protocol Review Committee guidelines for preparing clinical trial protocols and records are exemplary. Furthermore, one should mention the vast facilities of the Data Center of the EORTC. This Data Center, managed by Dr. M. Staquet and his efficient team, handles information received from different groups of researchers and represents a most remarkable resource for data processing and analysis. The aims of the EORTC regarding the improvement of cooperative clinical trials and the promotion of closer collaboration between clinicians and basic scientists correspond exactly to the objectives of the newly created training programs in Spain.

In view of the great potential of the Spanish Hospital System, it is hoped that we will rapidly enlarge our participation in the activities of the EORTC and adopt its standards and protocols for the conduct of clinical trials. A permanent willingness to cooperate and constant mutual incentives, both within and between hospitals, must be further encouraged and maintained.

CLINICAL TRIALS

Results from phase I and phase II clinical trials regarding drugs recently introduced into human medical care are presented and discussed in this volume. Some data are promising, others are less so, but they all indicate the obstinacy with which medical science is progressively trying to defeat cancer by means of trials, tests, and studies at all levels.

Phase II clinical trials must be numerous and must be performed according to the strictest standards to properly select optimal treatment options for phase III trials. Thus it should be possible to prevent patients from being unnecessarily exposed to therapeutic approaches that are ineffective or toxic. Moreover, data obtained from phase II trials are those providing the most useful information for setting up models or programs of drug associations that may have a synergistic action on certain tumors and, at the same time, decreased toxic effects.

Among the drugs that have successfully passed phase I and phase II trials and are now in clinical use, cisplatin has achieved the most promising results. This compound has had a significant influence on the increase of complete remission rates achieved in testicular and other genitourinary tumors. Epipodophyllotoxins are promising for the treatment of leukemia, lymphomas, and some selected solid tumors. At present, VP-16-213 is probably the best known agent available against small cell lung cancer; VM-26 has been increasingly incorporated into combination chemotherapy regimens for a number of tumor types. Two other drugs with promise are acridinylamino methanesulphon-*m*-anisidide (AMSA) and phosphonacetyl-L-aspartate (PALA), although these agents are still at an early stage of study.

The development of analogs of chemical structures with known antitumor activity represents a line of research attempting to reduce side effects and to increase antitumor activity relative to the parent compound. Additional trials with vindesine, a new vinca alkaloid derivative, are awaited with great expectations. Among the analogs of adriamycin, initial results have been favorable with 4'-epiadriamycin, aclacinomycin A, and demethoxyadriamycin. Platinum derivatives are also being examined and might represent a second generation of active agents in a new class of antitumor drugs.

Finally, I would like to emphasize a very important factor, the combined or sequential use of the three basic weapons available at the moment against cancer—surgery, radiation therapy, and chemotherapy. This approach, together with better knowledge of neoplastic diseases, has been instrumental in current therapeutic progress. The second section of this volume is devoted to the analysis of results obtained with combined modalities. This information will undoubtedly be immensely useful in our daily struggle against malignant diseases.

J. M. Segovia Arana, M.D.
Universidad Autónoma
Madrid, Spain

New Approaches in Cancer Therapy,
edited by H. Cortés Funes and M. Rozencweig.
Raven Press, New York © 1982.

Approach to Phase I Trials in Cancer Patients

Marcel Rozencweig, Pierre Dodion, Claude Nicaise,
Martine Piccart, and Yvon Kenis

Department of Chemotherapy, Institut Jules Bordet, Centre des Tumeurs de l'Université Libre de Bruxelles, Laboratoire d'Investigation Clinique H. J. Tagnon, Brussels, Belgium

Current anticancer chemotherapeutic agents lack specificity and produce a variety of toxic effects at therapeutic doses. As single drug therapy, these agents are commonly given in man at, or near, the maximum tolerated dose (MTD) for a specified mode of administration. This is particularly important for meaningful early clinical trials aimed at screening for antitumor activity. However, definition of this MTD may vary greatly according to individual investigator criteria, type of disease to be treated, and quality of supportive care available.

When a new agent is introduced into clinical trials, its MTD must be determined prior to evaluating its anticancer activity. This objective is reached in phase I trials, at given schedules and routes of administration, by progressive increments of an initial dose extrapolated from animal data. These phase I trials are also designed to characterize toxic effects at increasing dose levels and to identify dose-limiting factors. Their ultimate purpose is to define adequate modalities of drug administration and follow-up for exploring therapeutic efficacy in subsequent trials. These variables should be determined at least for ambulatory patients with solid tumors. Concomitant pharmacokinetic investigations might be helpful to achieve these goals.

Phase I trials are carried out to answer important, but limited, toxicologic and pharmacologic questions. They should not be expected to provide definitive information on rates of toxic effects, long-term toxic effects, and tolerance to prolonged treatment. These data are obtained in phase II and III trials, which also identify rare toxic effects with greater probability. Although focus is on toxicologic information, phase I trials must always be conducted with therapeutic intent. Any hints of antitumor effect are encouraging for further investigation, but apparent lack of activity in these early trials should not prevent phase II trials from being initiated (30): diseases treated in phase I studies are largely refractory to conventional chemotherapy, small numbers of patients are entered per tumor types, and some of these may not be truly assessable for activity because of suboptimal dosage, insufficient treatment duration, and/or lack of clearly evaluable lesions.

Some particular aspects of phase I trials deserve special consideration. These selected points are discussed here.

RELEVANCE OF QUALITATIVE TOXICOLOGY DATA FOR PHASE I CLINICAL TRIALS

The largest analysis of the relationship between experimental and clinical qualitative findings was conducted retrospectively by Schein et al. (24) and involved 25 anticancer drugs with preclinical evaluations in dogs and monkeys. The data suggested that all serious organ system toxicities were well predicted with the possible exception of central nervous system and dermal toxicity. However, a high percentage of false-positive predictions was encountered, and this overprediction was ascribed to the administration of severely toxic or lethal doses as well as more extensive toxicologic evaluations in the animals. It could also be somewhat related to the lack of critical interpretation of the meaning and weight of some symptoms and biological signs.

Animal toxicology investigations are carried out to alert the clinician to potential hazards of the drugs (23). If relevant, these investigations would be most helpful for unusual toxic effects. However, the prediction of a rare event is, obviously, less likely to be correct than a prediction of a common event. Using a Bayesian approach, the variability of this likelihood may be estimated in relation to the frequency of the predicted event (5).

Suppose that the occurrence of a particular toxic effect T is determined in animals and in humans for 100 drugs. Suppose that 50 drugs produce T in humans, whereas 40 of these and 20 of the remaining drugs produce T in animals (Table 1). Animal models are considered here as testing the hypothesis that drugs do not induce this effect T in man. The rate of false-positive findings, or α error, is then 40% (20/50) and the rate of false-negative findings, or β error, is 20% (10/50). The proportion *(p)* of drugs inducing T in man may be viewed as the *a priori* probability (50/100) that an individual drug will produce T in man and is defined here as the prevalence of T. One may then determine the *a posteriori* probability (PV^+) that a drug producing T in animals will also produce T in humans (40/60) and the *a posteriori* probability (PV^-) that a drug that does not produce T in animals will not produce T in humans (30/40).

The following formulas give the relationship between PV^+ or PV^- and p, α, and β (5):

$$PV^+ = \frac{p\,(1 - \beta)}{p\,(1 - \beta) + \alpha\,(1 - p)}; PV^- = \frac{(1 - p)\,(1 - \alpha)}{(1 - p)\,(1 - \alpha) + p\beta}$$

Thus, for fixed α and β, as p tends to 0, PV^+ tends to 0 whereas PV^- tends to 1. The α and β errors truly characterize the experimental model and are not influenced by variations of p. In a meaningful predictive model, the probability of finding toxicity in man when present in animals must be greater than expected on the basis of what is known before doing the test. These requirements may be expressed as $PV^+ > p$ and, conversely, $PV^- > 1 - p$. This analysis is valid only for drugs

TABLE 1. *Example of distribution of drugs according to the occurrence of a toxic effect T in animals and in humans[a]*

T in animals	T in humans		
	Yes	No	Total
Yes	40	20	60
No	10	30	40
Total	50	50	100

[a]Prevalence (p) = 50/100; α error = 20/50; β error = 10/50; PV^+ = 40/60; PV^- = 30/40.

TABLE 2. *Probability (PV^+) of observing in man a toxic effect observed in the dog and the most sensitive of the dog and the monkey*

Organ system	Prevalence in man (%)	PV^+	
		Dog (%)	Dog + monkey (%)
Gastrointestinal	92	92 (25)[a]	92 (25)
Bone marrow	88	87 (23)	88 (25)
Liver	52	54 (24)	52 (25)
Renal	40	36 (22)	39 (23)
Cardiovascular	40	54 (13)	53 (17)
Neuromuscular	28	29 (21)	29 (21)
Integument	28	27 (11)	40 (15)
Injection site	24	31 (13)	31 (13)
Respiratory	20	20 (20)	17 (23)
Lymphoid	4	5 (19)	5 (20)

[a]( ) = Number of drugs. Prevalence is based on findings with 25 drugs.
Adapted from Schein et al. (24).

belonging to a homogeneous class of chemicals. This may be reasonably assumed with cytotoxic agents used in cancer chemotherapy and selected for clinical trials according to similar experimental criteria.

To illustrate these concepts, findings with the 25 anticancer drugs previously reported by Schein et al. (24) have been reanalyzed in terms of PV^+ values (20). Table 2 summarizes the corresponding clinical, chemical, and pathologic toxicology data by organ systems in the dog and the most sensitive species of the dog and the monkey (20). The relatively small number of drugs available for analysis allows only a rough estimate of the relevance to the clinical setting of toxicologic findings in animals. Nevertheless, a number of striking observations may be made.

Since the predictive value of a predictive test is dependent on the prevalence, the predictability will be relatively high for common toxicities to which all investigators are *a priori* already alerted, whereas this predictability will be relatively low for rare toxic effects. This relationship is well illustrated in Table 2.

Moreover, the available data seem to indicate that, overall, the predictive value of qualitative toxic effects in large animals is not significantly superior to a prediction entirely based on the prevalence of the toxic effects. Little variations in this prevalence should be expected as long as screening methods for selecting new drugs for cancer therapy remain unchanged.

Also of interest, findings are basically similar with data in the dog alone or with combined data in the dog and the monkey. Other species could be used to determine which organ systems are affected by drug toxicity. However, there is no reason to believe that this type of toxicologic data would then be more relevant for the human situation.

Whether drug-induced toxic effects are reversible, delayed, cumulative, manageable, or predictable in animals is likely to be of greater help for designing phase I trials than the mere determination of which organ systems are impaired (17). The utilization of rodents seems attractive to reach rapidly and accurately this objective (8), but additional research is needed to identify the most appropriate species for this purpose. Animal toxicology models are widely developed for specific classes of compounds based on clinical findings, e.g., cardiomyopathy model with anthracyclines or renal tubular function with platinum derivatives. Further work is also necessary to evaluate the potential of these models to select subsequent analogs for clinical use.

SELECTION OF PATIENTS

The human tumor-cloning assay proposed by Salmon et al. (22) might play a significant role in selecting drugs for individual patients. Current data suggest a striking correlation between *in vitro* and *in vivo* antitumor activity. Compiled results (Table 3) indicate that the α and the β errors of this predictive system are 9% (24/259) and 17.5% (7/40), respectively. According to a Bayesian analysis (see previous section), the *a posteriori* probability (PV^+) that a drug achieving activity *in vitro* will also achieve activity in patients varies directly with the prevalence *p*. In this example (Table 3), despite a very low value of *p* (40/299 or 13%), PV^+

TABLE 3. *Correlation between human tumor cloning assay and clinical response to chemotherapy*

	No. of patients		
	Response	Failure	Total
In vitro response	33	24	57
In vitro failure	7	235	242
	40	259	299

Data compiled from Salmon et al. (21) and Von Hoff (26).

(33/57) still approaches 60%. Thus, this assay might provide most useful information even in a population of patients with diseases largely refractory to chemotherapy. Conversely, as expected from the very low prevalence (40/299 or 13%), PV^- reaches high values, i.e., 235/242 or 97% (Table 3). However, lack of *in vitro* sensitivity to new drugs must be interpreted with caution since, generally, active species are not yet identified and optimal $C \times t$ values for *in vitro* drug exposure are still unknown. On the other hand, if conventional agents are used, absence or minimal cell kill *in vitro* might be an indication for clinical treatment with investigational regimens.

Promising findings reported with this assay require confirmation in prospective trials, and several technical problems remain to be solved. With current procedures, adequate *in vitro* cell growth for drug sensitivity testing may be obtained in one-half of the patients only (28), pointing to the need for substantially increasing the yield of this assay.

Eligibility criteria for phase I trials are set at a minimum. A distinction should be made between patients entered at the beginning of the trial and those in whom a recommended dose is proposed for phase II trials. Overall, the former population represents a less favorable selection of patients with particular respect to prior cytotoxic therapy, performance status, and, occasionally, impaired function of excretory organs. In principle, patients with these unfavorable pretreatment characteristics should not be denied the potential benefit of a new treatment; they may be eligible at initiation of the study. Lack of toxicity in these high-risk patients at a particular dose level is important to recognize when considering the magnitude of the next dose escalation. During the phase I trial, characteristics that interfere with drug tolerance are progressively identified and may become exclusion criteria for subsequent patients. In addition, intervals between retreatments may be lengthened during the trial if required by the time for recovery from toxic effects. This implies that, at higher dose levels, more prolonged survival expectancy may be needed to evaluate drug tolerance and to give time for allowing antitumor activity, if any. In the final analysis, interpretation of the dose-response relationship may be obscured by this continuous variability in eligibility criteria.

Whatever the dose level at entry, there are several important requirements for patient selection in a phase I study. All patients must have microscopically confirmed diagnosis of cancer. Initial trials should be restricted to patients with solid tumors. They should have a performance status on the Zubrod scale ≤3 (Table 4) and a life expectancy of at least 6 weeks. Survival may be difficult to estimate with accuracy in end-stage patients who are specially prone to develop intercurrent disease-related complications and who may recover with difficulty from drug-induced side effects. Based on the scanty data currently available (29), it seems advisable to carry out phase I trials separately in children and adults.

The disease may not, or no longer, be suitable for any form of known effective therapy. Patients must be off all previous anticancer therapy for at least 4 weeks (longer for nitrosoureas and mitomycin C) and have recovered from major toxic effects of prior treatment.

TABLE 4. *Performance status scale*

Karnofsky		Ecog-Zubrod	
Status	Scale	Scale	Status
Normal, no complaints	100	0	Normal activity
Able to carry on normal activities; minor signs or symptoms of disease	90	1	Symptoms, but nearly fully ambulatory
Normal activity with effort	80		
Cares for self; unable to carry on normal activity or to do active work	70	2	Some bed time, but needs to be in bed less than 50% of normal daytime
Requires occasional assistance, but able to care for most needs	60		
Requires considerable assistance and frequent medical care	50	3	Needs to be in bed more than 50% of normal daytime
Disabled; requires special care and assistance	40		
Severely disabled; hospitalization indicated though death not imminent	30	4	Unable to get out of bed
Very sick; hospitalization necessary; active supportive treatment necessary	20		
Moribund	10		
Dead	0		

Minimal hematologic requirements are commonly white blood cells (WBC) $\geq 4,000/mm^3$ and platelets $\geq 100,000/mm^3$. Hepatic and renal functions should be normal. There should be no organ dysfunction in a site of known or assumed toxic effects, e.g., cardiomyopathy for anthracyclines. Patients with rapid alteration of major organ functions should be excluded. Pregnancy and acute intercurrent complications are contraindictions to enter the trial.

DRUG SCHEDULE

The probable mechanism of action of the drug and its cell cycle specificity, schedule dependency in animal systems, and pharmacokinetic data are commonly used as rationales to select drug schedules for phase I trials. Practically, the relevance of these experimental data for defining the most appropriate schedule in man is often difficult to demonstrate. Convincing evidence of schedule dependency of activity is rather rare in man. This effect of the schedule has been recently suggested in a randomized trial comparing various modes of administration of VP-16-213 in small cell lung cancer (4). Thus, a significantly higher response rate was found when the drug was given orally for 3 consecutive days repeated weekly relative to the i.v. once-weekly schedule. Myelosuppression was similar in both treatment arms. In contrast, schedule dependency of toxicity has been frequently reported for early as well as chronic toxicity. This is well illustrated by the variable toxicity of adriamycin according to schedule. Initial experience indicated that a 10-fold decrease in the incidence of stomatitis could be obtained with a single-dose intermittent schedule as compared to repeated daily administrations (18). A more recent analysis of data generated by the cooperative groups in the United States confirmed that the probability of developing congestive heart failure with adriamycin was related to the total dose of drug administered and that a weekly dose schedule was associated with a significantly lower incidence of this cardiac effect than was the usually employed every 3-week schedule (27). Experience with ICRF-159 is also illustrative of the importance of the schedule (2). Following oral administration of this compound, toxicity was erratic with a single-dose schedule and became dose dependent with fractionated daily doses. This phenomenon was ascribed to a plateau in the intestinal absorption of the drug.

The single-dose intermittent schedule is often preferred, as an initial schedule, in phase I trials. Generally, it is most convenient for the patients, it provides the clearest drug evaluation, and, for identical number of dose escalation steps, it allows the fastest study completion. Investigation of additional schedules is particularly recommended if, at the initial schedule, disturbing nonhematologic factors such as CNS toxic effects are dose limiting. Practically, however, phase I studies are often undertaken concomitantly in different institutions and it is then advisable to investigate several schedules simultaneously.

STARTING DOSE

The starting dose of phase I clinical trials may not exceed the MTD and should be sufficiently high to avoid prolonged investigations at ineffective doses. Determination of the starting dose is essentially based on animal toxicology data, unless previous clinical experience is available.

Body surface area seems to correlate better with certain metabolic and excretory functions than body weight; moreover, it was shown that drug dosage could be more readily compared between species when doses were expressed on a mg/m^2 body surface basis than on a mg/kg basis (15). A detailed study was conducted by Freireich et al. (7) to compare quantitatively the toxicity of 18 anticancer agents in the mouse, rat, hamster, dog, monkey, and man. All animal species included in that analysis proved to be equally relevant for predicting the MTD in humans. Available dose schedules were converted to a uniform schedule of daily treatment for 5 consecutive days. After logarithmic transformation of the data, regression lines indicated a linear relationship between MTD in man, LD_{10} in rodents, and highest nonlethal dose in dogs or monkeys, respectively.

These observations were confirmed in subsequent retrospective analyses using additional anticancer agents (9,11,13) and provided the rationale for using a particular fraction of the MTD in the most sensitive of several species as a starting dose for initial clinical trials in man. The recommended fraction of the MTD on a mg/m^2 basis in the most susceptible animal has varied from ⅓ to ⅕ (7,12).

The suitability of this procedure seems related to the type of species selected for these determinations. In a study based on experimental data in the dog and the monkey, Homan showed that a prediction from the more sensitive species did not provide a significantly greater margin of safety than one of the species alone (11).

Using $\frac{1}{10}$ of the MTD in units of mg/m^2 in dog or monkey carried the same risk of 1% of exceeding the MTD in man whereas using the more sensitive species minimally decreased this risk to 0.5%. Using $\frac{1}{3}$ of the MTD, the risk was 10% with either species and 6% with the most sensitive.

One-third of the toxic dose low (TDL) in dog or monkey, whichever is lower, has been largely used as a starting dose in phase I clinical trials sponsored by the National Cancer Institute. The TDL has been defined as the lowest dose that produces drug-induced pathologic alterations in hematologic, chemical, clinical, or morphologic parameters; doubling the TDL produces no lethality (16). The toxic dose high (TDH) is also a dose that produces any of these alterations, but doubling this dose does produce lethality.

In a recent analysis (20), MTD in man was compared to LD$_{10}$ in mice and TDL in dogs. Twenty-one agents were included in this analysis. They were selected because experimental and clinical results were available at an identical schedule, allowing a direct comparison of the data without any extrapolation. Units were eventually converted from mg/kg to mg/m^2 (7). Actual figures were obtained from data on file with the Division of Cancer Treatment, National Cancer Institute.

The highest fraction of the experimental toxic dose levels that were still lower than the MTD in man for all drugs included in this analysis approximated $\frac{1}{6}$ LD$_{10}$ in the mouse and $\frac{1}{3}$ TDL in the dog. The data confirmed that these species were equally relevant for predicting MTD in man, at least when the entire group of drugs was considered. Thus, the ratios of MTD in man to $\frac{1}{6}$ LD$_{10}$ in the mouse and those of MTD in man to $\frac{1}{3}$ TDL in the dog fit very similar distribution curves. However, for individual drugs, the mouse and the dog provided markedly different information, as indicated by a large range (0.23 to 26.00 +) of the ratios of the LD$_{10}$ in the mouse to the TDL in the dog. These variable relationships suggested that a combination of data generated in both species could be useful for determining acceptable starting doses in man.

Various procedures could be advocated for this purpose. One might decide to base the decision on the most sensitive species and to select the lowest value of $\frac{1}{6}$ LD$_{10}$ in the mouse and $\frac{1}{3}$ TDL in the dog. Another approach consists of initiating clinical trials with a fraction of the LD$_{10}$ in the mouse, provided that the resulting dose is tolerated in the dog. If life-threatening or lethal toxicity is seen in the dog, the clinical dose would have to be calculated according to further toxicologic investigations in this species. With this approach the burden of routinely determining the TDL would no longer be necessary. One-tenth of the LD$_{10}$ in the mouse would seem generally adequate since this fraction does not exceed the TDH in the dog, at least with the drugs selected in this analysis.

On the average, there was no difference in terms of number of dose escalation steps in phase I clinical trials between (a) the selection of the lowest of either $\frac{1}{6}$ LD$_{10}$ in the mouse or $\frac{1}{3}$ TDL in the dog and (b) the selection of $\frac{1}{10}$ LD$_{10}$ in the mouse when this dose proves to be tolerated in the dog. With the rationales presently used to define a tolerated starting dose in man, it is unlikely that this starting dose could be set uniformly at a level significantly closer to the human MTD without increasing noticeably the risk of exceeding this human MTD.

Thus it would appear that, from a quantitative point of view, there is no great advantage in employing one species instead of another for predicting acceptable starting doses in man, at least when based on fractions of LD_{10}, TDL, or probably any other toxic dose level. It is clear that if the most sensitive species determines this starting dose in man, the greater the number of species, the lower the starting dose, and the greater the chance of starting below the MTD in man. However, a sufficiently low fraction of a specific toxic dose level in a single species (i.e., $\frac{1}{10}$ LD_{10} in the mouse, expressed as mg/m^2) proves equally satisfactory, especially if its relative safety is tested in another animal species. Although retrospective data should be interpreted with caution (10), it appears that the mouse can be a primary animal for quantitative toxicologic evaluation, particularly in view of the large number of animals that may be used in toxicology experiments.

DOSE ESCALATION SCHEME

Schneiderman initially discussed the value of progressively smaller dose increments, based on an inverted Fibonacci series, for phase I studies (25). The Fibonacci series is related to problems of cumulative growth and consists of a sequence of numbers in which the first two terms are 0 and 1 and each succeeding term is the sum of the two immediately preceding (0, 1, 1, 2, 3, 5, 8, 13, 21 . . .). Over the last few years, the escalation method most widely referred to has been the so-called idealized modified Fibonacci search scheme approach. This method uses successive percentage increases above the preceding dose level of 100, 67, 50, and 40, with subsequent increments of 30 to 35% (3). Goldsmith et al. suggested that a maximum of six escalation steps of such scheme would be required to reach the MTD for about 75% of the drugs with starting doses corresponding to 1/3 TDL in the dog (9). Actually, compliance with this escalation procedure has been highly flexible.

Once toxic levels are reached, further escalations should be based on specific findings at each level and on dose-response relationships. Practically, the main problem is with escalating doses within the nontoxic range. As might have been expected, the ratio of the LD_{90} to the LD_{10} in the mouse and that of the TDH to the TDL in the dog do not provide useful information: the former has no "physiologic" parallelism to the clinical situation, whereas the determination of TDH and TDL lacks accuracy (6). Safety of a rapid escalation procedure is connected with the availability of effective measures to control dose-limiting toxicity. Unfortunately, at this point, dose-limiting factors may not be predicted with sufficient accuracy (19,20), with the possible exception of analogs of already clinically investigated compounds. Continuous increments of 100% are probably possible with drugs achieving dose-limiting myelosuppression, which is most frequent. Thus, in a phase I trial with carminomycin in solid tumors (1), a steep dose-response relationship was found, and the highest dose tested was 22 mg/m^2 given as a single i.v. dose (Table 5). Currently, total doses per course of 60 mg/m^2 (12 $mg/m^2 \times 5$)

TABLE 5. *Carminomycin-induced leukopenia*

i.v. Dose (mg/m² q. 3 weeks)	No. of evaluable patients/No. of evaluable courses	Median nadir × 10⁹/1	
		Leukocytes (range)	Granulocytes (range)
12	1/2	2.9	1.9
15	4/5	4.35 (0.5–4.9)	2.8 (0.3–3.6)
18	5/6	2.9 (0.7–3.3)	1.8 (0.2–2.5)
20	6/11	1.75 (0.5–6.8)	1.0 (0.2–4.1)
22	6/7	1.1 (0.2–5.6)	0.5 (0.1–4.6)

TABLE 6. *Toxic effects of α-triglycidyl-s-triazinetrione*

i.v. Dose (mg/m² q. 2 weeks)	No. of patients/ No. of courses	No. of toxic patients	No. of patients with			
			Phlebitis	Nausea and vomiting	Leukopenia	Loss of hair
33	2/3	1		1		
66	3/4	1		1		
130	5/6	1			1	
260	3/3	1				1
400	3/3	2				2
600	3/3	3	2	2		
900	5/5	5	5	3	1	
1,350	4/5	4	4	3		
2,000	5/5	5	5	4	2	

are employed in acute leukemia with reversible myelosuppression (M. Malarme, M. Rozencweig, and P. Strijckmans, *unpublished data*). Although schedules and diseases are different in these studies, results suggest that doubling the initially defined MTD in solid tumors might still yield manageable toxicity.

In fact, safety in a phase I trial may not be so much dependent on the dose escalation per se, but on the availability of adequate treatment facilities and the care with which the study is conducted in selecting patients and in monitoring toxic manifestations. At Jules Bordet, we are prospectively evaluating a procedure consisting of initial escalations by increments of 100% (with starting doses = 1/10 LD_{10} in the mouse) followed by increments of 50% up to toxic levels. This is exemplified by our phase I study with α-triglycidyl-*s*-triazinetrione (Table 6) (14). This compound is a new alkylating agent that has shown attractive properties in experimental tumor models. In man, local phlebitis was dose limiting, with a single-dose schedule at doses that did not produce other dose-limiting toxic effects, thus preventing this schedule from being utilized for phase II studies. Four additional escalation steps, several more months of investigations, and a number of additional patients treated at ineffective doses would have been required to obtain the same result with an idealized modified Fibonacci search scheme approach.

As discussed above, entry of eligible, but poor-risk, patients at nontoxic dose levels might provide valuable information on the safety of the following escalation step. Identification of cumulative toxicity may also be useful for determining the next escalation, particularly when cumulation becomes rapidly apparent with repeated courses. The usefulness of this observation emphasizes the need for retreatments in phase I trials. In fact, all patients should be scheduled to receive at least 2 courses or 4 weeks of treatment, whichever is longer. Further characterization of this cumulative toxicity must be made at the MTD, but its full assessment is generally possible in phase II and III trials only.

Special attention should be paid to the possibility of cumulative or delayed toxicity in the light of animal toxicology investigations and clinical experience with analogs. In any event, retreatment should always be considered with caution, particularly in patients with decreasing general condition during the previous courses and, consequently, with potentially decreasing tolerance to therapy. It should be kept in mind that eligibility criteria must also be met for retreatment, specifically with respect to performance status, intercurrent complications, as well as hematologic, hepatic, and renal functions. Dose escalation in the same patient must be avoided after a previously toxic course; it could be allowed in patients experiencing nontoxic courses at a particular dose level if careful monitoring indicates reproducible individual tolerance and clear lack of cumulative and delayed effects at this dose level or lack of toxicity at the next higher dose level. Reentries at increasing doses may be important for therapeutic purposes and may yield useful toxicology information since patients can then serve as their own controls.

Optimally, only new and good-risk patients should be entered initially at new dose levels. Time intervals between entries must be appropriately defined. For the lower and nontoxic doses, 3 patients per dose are probably adequate, but as significant toxicity is demonstrated, at least 5 patients are usually evaluated at each level. Additional patients may be needed if there is a wide variation in the individual tolerance to the drug. This seems to occur frequently with drugs producing toxicity with a steep dose-response relationship (Table 5) (1).

Potential contributions of clinical pharmacology data to phase I trials may be substantial, although meaningful elucidation of the pharmacokinetics of a new drug may require prolonged periods of time. Determination of drug disposition and .metabolism, as well as correlation of toxicity with plasma drug levels, may profoundly influence the design and the mechanics of these trials. These aspects have been nicely and extensively reviewed by Woolley and Schein (31) and will not be further discussed here.

CONCLUSION

The design of phase I trials should be essentially guided by the prime need for determining rapidly and safely the method of drug administration in a population for whom phase II trials are planned. Interim data are required only to the extent that they allow faster and safer completion of the study. It seems difficult to provide investigators with standardized procedures, and this chapter, actually, raises more problems than it answers questions. The complexities of phase I trials stem largely from the necessary flexibility in the conduct of the trial and from the modifications that may be permanently introduced in the study protocol, based on the continuous flow of information and a correct interpretation of the data generated by the trial.

Specific ethical problems of phase I trials make these undertakings even more difficult, especially at nontoxic doses where only a placebo effect may be obtained and at the highest doses where patients with short life expectancy may require aggressive supportive care for severe toxic effects. Rationales for introducing new drugs into clinical trials represent another aspect of these problems, and, in this regard, full evaluation of the potential of the human tumor cloning assay is awaited with great expectations.

Over the last few years, phase I trials have been characterized by increasing sophistication. The approach to phase I trials has been slowly but continuously evolving, and it may be anticipated that guidelines outlined in this chapter will have to be revised in the near future.

ACKNOWLEDGMENTS

The authors acknowledge the work of Geneviève Decoster in the preparation of this manuscript.

This work was supported in part by contract NIH NO1-CM 53840 from the National Cancer Institute (NCI, Bethesda, Maryland) and by grant n° 3.4535.79 of the Fonds de la Recherche Scientifique Médicale (FRSM, Brussels, Belgium).

REFERENCES

1. Abele, R., Rozencweig, M., Body, J.-J., Bedogni, P., Reich, S. D., Crooke, S. T., Lenaz, L., and Kenis, Y. (1980): Carminomycin (NSC-180024): A phase I study. *Eur. J. Cancer*, 16:1,555–1,559.
2. Bellet, R. E., Rozencweig, M., Von Hoff, D. D., Penta, J. S., Wasserman, T. H., and Muggia, F. M. (1977): ICRF-159: Current status and clinical prospects. *Eur. J. Cancer*, 13:1,293–1,298.
3. Carter, S. K., Selawry, O., and Slavik, M. (1977): Phase I clinical trials. *Natl. Cancer Inst. Monogr.*, 45:75–80.
4. Cavalli, F., Sonntag, R. W., Jungi, F., Senn, H. J., and Brunner, K. W. (1978): VP-16-213 monotherapy for remission induction of small cell lung cancer: A randomized trial using three dosage schedules. *Cancer Treat. Rep.*, 62:473–475.
5. Chiang, C. L., Hodges, J. L., and Yerushalmy, J. (1956): Statistical problems in medical diagnoses. In: *Proceedings of the Third Berkeley Symposium on Mathematical Statistics and Probability, Vol. 4*, edited by J. Neyman, pp. 121–148. University of California Press, Berkeley.
6. Creaven, P. J., and Mihich, E. (1977): The clinical toxicity of anticancer drugs and its prediction. *Semin. Oncol.*, 4:147–163.
7. Freireich, E. J., Gehan, E. A., Rall, D. P., Schmidt, L. H., and Skipper, H. E. (1966): Quantitative comparison of toxicity of anticancer agents in mouse, rat, hamster, dog, monkey, and man. *Cancer Chemother. Rep.*, 50:219–244.
8. Goldin, A., Rozencweig, M., Guarino, A. M., and Schein, P. (1979): Quantitative and qualitative prediction of toxicity from animals to human. In: *Controversies in Cancer. Design of Trials and Treatment*, edited by H. J. Tagnon and M. J. Staquet, pp. 83–104. Masson Publishing USA, Inc., New York.

The synthesis has been described by Keller-Juslen et al. (60). With the chemical reagents of 4,6-O-ethylidene-2,3-di-O-acetyl-β-D-glucotoxin, in the presence of boron trifluoride etherate, a molecule is formed that, with application of $Zn(OCOCH_3)_2$ and $Na(OCOCH_3)_2$ and reduction with Pd-C, gives up VP-16 (Fig. 2).

VP-16 is not very soluble in water and can be diluted only in a detergent mixture of dimethylsulfoxide (DMSO) and Tween 80 or in a mixture of polyethylene glycol 300, ethanol, and Tween 80.

For clinical use, VP-16 is supplied in vials for injections and in capsules and liquid for oral administration. The vials for injectable use contain 100 mg of VP-16, 400 mg of Tween 80, 3.25 mg of polyethylene 300, 10 mg of anhydrous citric acid, and up to 5 cc of absolute alcohol. The preparation is not stable in glucose solutions and has to be diluted in sodium chloride solutions.

ACTION

Although the modes of action of VP-16 have not been sufficiently clarified, there are substantial data on the subject.

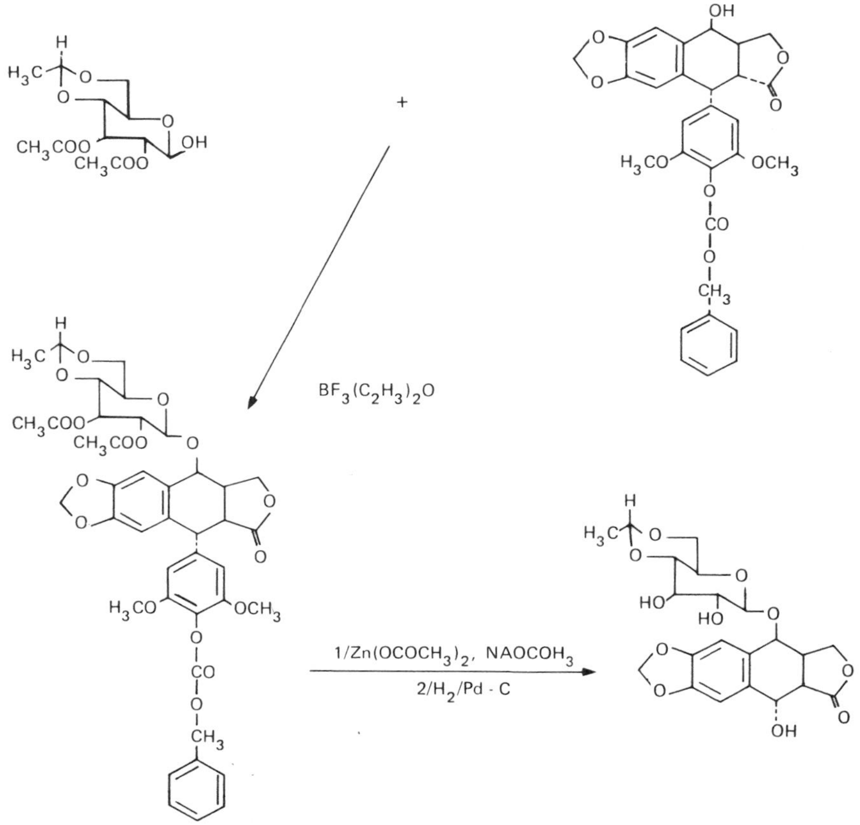

FIG. 2.   Chemical steps in the synthesis of VP-16-213.

Grieder et al. (46) experimented with a transplantable murine mastocytoma cell line and observed that the VP-16 withheld cells in their G_2 phase. VP-16 therefore differs in its action from other vegetal derivatives (colchicine, vincristine, etc.) that act as typical mitotic stoppers. Treatment with VP-16 reduced the mitotic ratio and stops the multiplication of the cells, but the amounts of deoxyribonucleic acid (DNA), ribonucleic acid (RNA), and proteins in the cells keep increasing, which suggests that the drug does not obstruct the way for cells through the S phase (32,62,69,97).

Loike and Horwitz (65) investigated the inclusion of nucleosides in HeLa cells treated with VP-16, and observed that the drug was capable of inhibiting, although in a reversible way, the incorporation of uridine, thymidine, adenosine, guanosine, and leucine, which would indicate an action on the synthesis of DNA, RNA, and proteins. Using alkaline sucrose gradients of radioactive DNA, Loike and Horwitz (66) observed that, in HeLa cells treated with VP-16, the DNA of high molecular weight changed to DNA of low molecular weight, which they interpreted as breaks in the DNA molecule induced by the VP-16. This effect is reversible, suppressing the cytostatic action on the cells, which suggests that they are single-stranded breaks, as double-stranded breaks are rarely repaired (99).

PHARMACOKINETICS

Creavan and Allen (26,27), using VP-16 marked with tritium, investigated the pharmacokinetic aspects of the cytostatic agent. A dose of 220 mg/m^2 was applied on 4 patients, and 290 mg/m^2 on another 5 patients, via i.v. in 1-hr perfusion. The plasma decay fitted a biexponential equation. Its half-life was 11.5 hr; VP-16 is rapidly cleared from the blood. The mean volume of distribution is 29% of the body weight. Seventy-two hr after its administration, 44% of the drug is detected in the urine (29% as such and 15% as metabolites of which the most important is the 4-demethylepipodophyllic acid-9-(4,6-O-ethylidene-β-D-glucopyranoside).The other main elimination tract, the gall bladder, allows the detection of 2 to 16% of fecal substances of the plasmatic levels (6).

Renal clearing of VP-16 takes six times as long as that of the VM-26, which indicates different degrees of affinity to the proteins. Approximately 74% of the drug can be detected associated with serous proteins, accumulations of etoposide of 10 μg/ml (5).

Due to its physicochemical characteristics, its low molecular weight, and its liposolubility, VP-16 penetrates the hematoencephalic barrier. Geran et al. (44) pointed out that VP-16 was effective against mouse ependymona implanted intra-cerebrally. The cytostatic levels in spinal fluid vary from 1 to 10% of the administered doses from 2 to 26 hr after administration.

Approximately 50% of VP-16 administered orally, in either liquid or capsule form, is absorbed (13).

IN VITRO AND ANIMAL ANTITUMOR ACTIVITY

VP-16 has shown a capacity to detain cell growth in culture (46,92). When 1 to 10 μg of VP-16 per ml are added to the culture, the cell growth is detained after 1.5 hr. Stäehlin (92) observed that the LD_{50} for the P815 mastocytome is 0.046 μg/ml whereas for the HeLa it is 0.14 μg/ml.

VP-16 is active in Ehrlich ascites, sarcoma 37 and 180, Walker carcinosarcoma, and in a variety of murine leukemias (P815, P1534, and L1210) (30,84,92). Its activity in the 1210 leukemia depends on the way in which it is administered. If applied in 3-hr intervals for 24 hr, VP-16 is considerably more active than when applied at other intervals. In experiments made with this type of leukemia, VP-16 has been shown to be synergistic with Ara C (83), cyclophosphamide and 1,3,bis(2-chloroethyl)-1-nitrosourea (BCNU) (30,75), and cis-platinum (67,86).

The lethal dose 50 for the mouse, rat, and rabbit is 118, 68, and 78 mg/kg, respectively (92). Subacute toxicity was investigated in monkeys (8,52,84). Several doses varying between 0.4 and 3.6 mg/kg were applied i.v. during 4 weeks. The animals on which a cytostatic agent had been applied presented hematological toxicity (anemia, leukopenia) as well as gastrointestinal (GI) and hepatic disorders.

DOSE SCHEDULES

The i.v. doses of VP-16 used in the phase 1 tests varied from 45 mg/m² to 290 mg/m² (28,75), depending on whether the applications were made daily or weekly. The dose variation for both oral forms depended on the therapeutic rest intervals interrupted by each therapeutic treatment.

No interval or form of administration of the drug has been proven better than another. At present, the 120 to 200 mg/m² dose is recommended for 3 to 5 days, followed by a resting period of 4 to 14 days. The patient must have a full stomach, and the global dose must not exceed 650 mg/m² per series. The dose for intravenous application varies from 60 to 120 mg/m² per day for 5 days with a free interval of 14 days (34). For i.v. administration, VP-16 must be diluted in a physiological saline solution of 250 cc and given over a period of 30 min. If this form is used, the total dose recommended per course is approximately half of the oral dose.

The usual number of courses prior to the evaluation of the results is three to four.

TOXICITY

Hematological

Leukopenia and thrombocytopenia are the phenomena associated with the depressing effect of VP-16 on the bone marrow (63,71,73). The former is much more frequent than the latter and is usually apparent after 8 to 10 days. Thrombocytopenia, if it occurs, appears 10 to 12 days after the application of the drug. Both disorders can be completely cured in 14 to 20 days. No cases of cumulative toxicity have been described, and the few cases of sepsis reported were in hypertreated patients.

The degree of medullary depression is similar in oral and venous applications. Chard et al. (24) applied the cytostatic in doses of less than 100 mg/m² per day during 5 days and observed no toxicity, although in doses of 125 to 150 mg/m² per day during 5 days, he observed a moderate medullary toxicity.

Cavalli et al. (20) investigated the effect of three different doses of VP-16, applied in different forms: (a) 250 mg/m², i.v., weekly; (b) 550 mg/m², oral, 3 days/week; and (c) 850 mg/m², oral, 5 days every 2 to 3 weeks. The toxicity was similar in the three groups. Of the 47 patients to which the cytostatic was applied, 71% presented leukopenia and 23% presented thrombocytopenia. Both disorders were reversible.

Gastrointestinal Disorders

GI disorders (nausea, vomiting, and, to a lesser degree, diarrhea) occur in approximately 25% of the patients treated with VP-16, more commonly with oral administration and large doses. With the use of capsules, there are fewer digestive reactions than with the drinkable vials, as the unpleasant taste of the drug is diminished. In any case, these disorders are easily controlled by prescribing antiemetic medication.

Another GI effect, of little importance, is anorexia.

Alopecia

Twenty-two to 93% of the patients present some degree of alopecia, depending mainly on the frequency and quantity of the administered doses.

Miscellaneous

The following disorders have been noticed, although with greater rarity:

1. Hypotension following rapid i.v. administration (less than 30 min), which disappears when the perfusion is slowed down (20,25,28).

2. Fever (38,93).

3. Chills (58).

4. Severe wheezing and bronchospasm following rapid administration, which ceases as soon as the infusion is withdrawn and antihistaminics are applied (93).

5. In relation with oral administration, cases of stomatitis have been described (13,42,48).

6. A case of generalized erythema (101) and a case of urticariform erythema localized in radiated areas 3 weeks before applying VP-16 (43) have been observed.

7. Cecil et al. (21) observed 2 patients that presented an increase of alkaline phosphatase. The hepatic biopsy showed variations compatible with medicamentose toxicity. This makes VP-16 contraindicated in patients suffering severe hepatic insufficiency.

8. Peripheral neuropathy is observed in 10 to 20% of treated cases (75).

9. In some patients the presence of palpitations and subexternal dysphoria has been noticed, but these cases are not well documented.

10. A 27-year-old patient suffered a myocardium attack in which the inducement of the cardiomyopathy was attributed to VP-16 (87). Mosijczuk (70) describes the case of 2 young children with leukemia, in whom previous VP-16 therapeutics apparently constituted a predisposing factor to cardiomyopathy through antracyclines administered as a second therapeutic option.

CLINICAL ACTIVITY

The clinical activity of VP-16, in both monotherapic regimes and in various combinations, has been investigated through several phase 2 and 3 investigations over the last 8 years. The effectiveness of the cytostatic agent seems to be centered mainly on acute myelocytic leukemia (AML), lymphomas, anaplastic bronchopulmonary carcinoma of small cells, and, to a lesser degree, germinal tumors of the testicle and Hodgkin's disease. A summary of the relative aspects of the reaction of various tumors when treated with VP-16 follows (see also Tables 1–4).

Lymphomas

In the initial investigations, VP-16 was active in non-Hodgkin lymphomas and in Hodgkin's disease. There have been few complete remissions produced by the

TABLE 1. *VP-16-213: Clinical activity in hematological neoplasms*

Condition	No. of patients	CR (*N*)	PR (*N*)	R (%)	Refs.
Lymphoma	135	2	41	31	21,24,38,42,45,55,57,68,81
Hodgkin's disease	71	0	11	15	21,24,38,76,82
ALL[a]	29	1	3	14	16,24,38,68,83
AML	158	19	19	24	16,17,24,33,38,41,53,68,74,78,82,91
Myelomonocytic AL	54	15	4	41	16,24,38,68,82

[a]ALL = Acute lymphoblastic leukemia.

TABLE 2. *VP-16-213 in SCLC*

Refs.	No. of patients	R (*N*)	R (%)
Jungi and Senn (58)	16	5	31
Eagan et al. (35)	16	7	44
Cohen et al. (25)	16	4	25
Hansen et al. (48)	40	20	50
Cavalli et al. (20)	56	23	41
Tucker et al. (93)	47	24	51
Brunner and Jungi (12)	86	35	41
Nissen et al. (76)	20	2	10
Total	297	120	40

TABLE 3. *Polichemotherapy studies in SCLC*

Refs.	Schedule	No. of patients	R (N)	R (%)
Aisner et al. (3)	VP-16 + doxorubicin + cyclophosphamide ± MER[a]	27	21	78
Cavalli et al. (14)	VP-16 + vincristine + methotrexate + cyclophosphamide	11	6	56
Eagan et al. (35)	VP-16 + cyclophosphamide	12	6	50
Broder et al. (11)	VP-16 + cyclophosphamide + procarbazine	14	13	93
Dombernowsky et al. (29)	VP-16 + doxorubicin	73	60	90
Schmieder et al. (88)	VP-16 + cyclophosphamide; VP-16 + doxorubicin	10 14	1 7	10 50
Sierocki et al. (89)	VP-16 + cisplatinum	21 (LD)[b] 17 (ED)[c]	21 15	100 88
Estapé et al. (39)	VP-16 + cyclophosphamide	6	4	66
Aisner and Wiernik (4)	VP-16 + cyclophosphamide + doxorubicin ± MER	32	31	97
Estapé et al. (40)	VP-16 + cyclophosphamide;	16	12	75
	VP-16 + cyclophosphamide + doxorubicin;	7	5	71
	VP-16 + cyclophosphamide + methotrexate	12	6	50
Vincent et al. (98)	VP-16 + doxorubicin + vincristine	46	38	83
Cortes et al. (personal communication)	VP-16 + cyclophosphamide + cisplatinum	24	15	62.5

[a]MER = Methanol-extraction residue of BCG.
[b]LD = Limited disease.
[c]ED = Extended disease.

TABLE 4. *Experience with VP-16 + cyclophosphamide in non-SMLC*

Schedule + ref.	No. of patients	R (N)	R (%)
VP-16 + cyclophosphamide (39)	24	15	62
VP-16 + cyclophosphamide (40)	14	4	28
VP-16 + cyclophosphamide + doxorubicin (40)	23	3	13
VP-16 + cyclophosphamide + methotrexate (40)	18	5	28

cytostatic, and the duration of the response was generally short. The cumulative effectiveness of VP-16 on lymphomas varies approximately from 30% in cases of histiocytic lymphoma to only 15% in cases of Hodgkin's disease. In cases of mixed or lymphocytic lymphoma, it is less effective.

VP-16 is not indicated as monotherapy, except in cases in which the first therapeutic options have failed. It is indicated in polychemotherapeutic treatment in experimental combinations for the development of guidelines that do not present any cross-resistance and in patients presenting a relapse in the primary treatments. At present, some groups are investigating the possibility of VP-16 as coadjuvant in the prolongation of the free interval of relapse in patients with a positive response to the conventional chemotherapy (80).

A few "complete responses" (CR) have been communicated in cases of mycosis fungoides. The investigations are based on 7 patients, and it is necessary to wait for the publication of further reports to determine the role VP-16 plays in such a process (56).

O'Connell et al. (77) obtained a 33% positive response (PR) in 15 patients suffering from previously treated lymphoma, with a combination of VP-16, doxorubicin, and prednisone.

Leukemias

The response rate of VP-16 was 24% in patients with AL, but it had a greater effectiveness (41% PR) in cases with monocytic acute leukemia (AML) (38). Mathe et al. (68) investigated 5 patients, 3 with monocytic AL, and 2 with myelomonocytic AL, all presenting a CR. The 2 patients with myelomonocytic AL showing CR had proved resistant to previous therapy with ARA C. VP-16 does not seem to act against acute lymphoblastic leukemia (ALL), as only 14% of the patients responded to the treatment. The tests were only made on a few cases, however. In cases of chronic myelomonocytic leukemia, a certain degree of activity of VP-16 has been observed (16,42,45).

Various investigations have been made with polichemotherapic treatment in cases of AML, comparing VP-16 with other drugs (96). Since these are effective agents in this disease, it is difficult to evaluate suitably the role VP-16 plays in the effectiveness of the mentioned treatment. As with the lymphomas, it seems necessary to research the role of VP-16 in combination of drugs in further investigative phases of the process of leukemia.

Lymphohistiocytic Reticulosis

Ambruso et al. (7) treated 2 patients suffering from lymphohistiocytic reticulosis with VP-16. Both presented hyperlipidemia associated with the process of this uncommon disease. Both patients had remission of their disease and a resolution of the hyperlipidemia.

Small Cell Lung Carcinoma

VP-16 is the most effective agent against small cell lung carcinomas (SCLC), with a PR in 40% of the cases. (See Table 2.)

Cavalli et al. (20) investigated different doses and forms of application in SCLC cases, observing that the ideal application form of the cytostatic agent is the oral one, more precisely, the drinkable vial. Although the number of patients that respond to the treatment is high, complete remissions are very few. At the same time, the response is usually maintained for only a short period of time in most of the tests.

Nevertheless, Tucker et al. (93) treated 47 cases of SCLC with VP-16 (60 mg/m^2, i.v. daily for 5 days and subsequently twice weekly, at the same dose, in drinkable vials). Twenty-three patients had not been previously treated and the rest had been submitted to radiotherapy and/or chemotherapy. Fifty-one percent responded positively to the treatment. The overall median survival was 225 days.

Due to its great effectiveness in a monotherapic regime, VP-16 in combination has been amply evaluated (Table 3). Most of the combinations used presented a large number of PR. Cyclophosphamide and adriamycin are the cytostatics generally used (10,22); recently, the drug cis-platinum has also been used and it has been described as acting synergistically with VP-16 (67).

Cortes et al. treated 24 patients suffering from SCLC, combining VP-16 with cyclophosphamide and cis-platinum *(personal communication)*. The response level was 58.5%, with 6 CR (25%) and 8 PR (33.3%), thus enforcing the idea that response is better in patients with a limited disease than in disseminated cases.

Our group (39,40) investigated the effectiveness of combinations of VP-16 and cyclophosphamide through four successive records. In our experience, this combination presents great effectiveness and, at the same time, an admissible toxicity. The results were not improved in any way by adding either adriamycin or methotrexate.

Other Histopathological Types

The level of response for the rest of cellular types affecting the lung is much lower (36,85). In cases of squamous cell carcinoma, 20% of the patients responded to treatment, whereas in adenocarcinoma or large-cell carcinoma only 13% of patients responded to treatment. In our investigations (39,40), in which the usefulness of the combination of VP-16 and cyclophosphamide was investigated, patients affected by these tumors were included. The results obtained are shown in the Table 4.

CNS

Although the cytostatic agent penetrates the hematoencephalic barrier, contrary to the action of its congener VM-26, VP-16 is not effective in tumors of the CNS (76).

Head and Neck Cancer

In the initial investigations made with VP-16, no PR was observed in head and neck tumors. This was recently confirmed by Nissen et al. (76). In 24 patients treated with VP-16, only 1 PR, 3 improvements, and 2 stabilized cases were observed.

Breast Cancer

The phase II investigations in breast cancer did not show any effectiveness of VP-16, as only 5% of the patients responded. They were, however, patients in whom the disease had spread amply and who had undergone polytreatments (1). It would seem that VP-16 in breast cancer has to be combined with other drugs, in order to find treatments that do not present cross-resistance to conventional therapies. Van Echo et al. (95) treated 15 patients with breast cancer that had already spread with a combination of VP-16 and adriamycin. They had all been previously treated with a combination that contained an alkylating agent, methotrexate, 5-fluorouracil ± vincristine and ± prednisone. Two patients showed CR (13%) and 4 showed PR (27%). This indicates the effectiveness of the combination of VP-16 and adriamycin and, more important, the fact that no cross-resistance was present with the conventional therapy.

Gastrointestinal Cancer

In GI cancer, VP-16 is not effective. Of 140 patients with colorectal cancer treated, only 6 showed objective response superior to 50% (4.5%) (31,76,79). Patients who had GI cancer in other areas responded better to therapy with VP-16 than those with colorectal cancer. Of 41 patients, 4 responded positively.

Hepatoma

The number of hepatoma patients studied is low, although the fact that some PR with VP-16 (18,79) has been found encourages further investigation of this drug in primitive hepatic carcinoma.

Genitourinary Tract

VP-16 has only presented activity in germinal testicular tumors or other localized tumors. The other neoplasms of this type do not respond, or do so only very little, to therapy with this cytostatic agent (47).

The experience with germinal tumors, although not extensive, shows that VP-16 is a promising drug (15); therefore, tests are being carried out based on the combination of VP-16 and cis-platinum, including adriamycin and bleomycin. The results have been encouraging. Williams et al. (100) treated 83 patients with VP-16 alone or in combination with cis-platinum, bleomycin, and, frequently, adriamycin. Although they had all undergone previous therapy, 14 patients presented CR and 15 presented PR.

Melanoma

Melanoma is a tumor that does not respond to therapy with VP-16 (2). Only in work done by EORTC (38) and us *(unpublished data)* has a slight PR been observed: 1 of 11 and 2 of 13 patients, respectively.

Miscellaneous

In phase II investigations carried out to date, patients suffering from neoplasms of other body areas, such as the esophagus, sarcoma of soft parts, neuroblastoma, and Wilms' tumor, have been studied (37,72,90). The number of patients treated is small and does not allow the extraction of any valid conclusions. Further investigations should be done on these sorts of tumors.

REFERENCES

1. Ahmann, D. L., Bisel, H. F., Eagan, R. T., Edmonson, J. H., Hahn, R. G., O'Connell, M. J., and Frytak, S. (1976): Phase II evaluation of VP-16-213 (NSC-141540) and cytembena (NSC-104801) in patients with advanced breast cancer. *Cancer Treat. Rep.*, 60:633–635.
2. Ahmann, D. L., Bisel, H. F., Edmonson, J. H., Hahn, R. G., O'Connell, M. J., and Frytak, S. (1976): Phase II study of VP-16-213 versus dianhydrogalactitol in patients with metastatic malignant melanoma. *Cancer Treat. Rep.*, 60:1,681–1,682.
3. Aisner, J., Esterhay, R. J., Jr., and Wiernik, P. H. (1977): Chemotherapy vs chemoimmunotherapy for small-cell carcinoma of the lung. *Proc. Am. Assoc. Cancer Res. and ASCO*, 18:310.
4. Aisner, J., and Wiernik, P. H. (1980): Chemotherapy versus chemoimmunotherapy for small-cell undifferentiated carcinoma of the lung. *Cancer*, 46:2,543–2,549.
5. Allen, L. M., and Creaven, P. J. (1975): Comparison of the human pharmacokinetics of VM-26 and VP-16-213, two antineoplastic epipodophyllotoxin glucopyranoside derivatives. *Eur. J. Cancer*, 11:697–707.
6. Allen, M. L., Marks, C., and Creaven, P. J. (1976): 4'-(Demethylepipodophyllic acid-9-(4,6-O-ethylidene-β-D-glucopyranoside). The major urinary metabolite of VP-16-213 in man. *Proc. Am. Assoc. Cancer Res. and ASCO*, 17:6.
7. Ambruso, D. R., Hays, T., Zwartjes, N. J., Tubergen, D. G., and Favara, B. E. (1980): Successful treatment of lymphohistiocytic reticulosis with phagocytosis with epipodophyllotoxin VP-16-213. *Cancer*, 45:2,516–2,520.
8. Arnold, A. M. (1979): Podophyllotoxin derivative VP-16-213. *Cancer Chemother. Pharmacol.*, 3:71–80.
9. Bentley, R. (1861): New American remedies. I. Podophyllum peltatum. *Pharmacol. J. Trans.*, 3:456–464.
10. Broder, L. E., Selawry, O. S., Bagnell, S. P., Silverman, M. A., and Charyulu, K. N. (1978): A controlled clinical trial testing two non-cross-resistant chemotherapy regimens in small-cell carcinoma of the lung. *Proc. Am. Assoc. Cancer Res. and ASCO*, 19:71.
11. Broder, L. E., Selawry, O. S., and Johnson, M. K. (1979): Treatment of small-cell carcinoma (SCC) of the lung utilizing mutually non-cross-resistant chemotherapy regimens. *Proc. Am. Assoc. Cancer Res. and ASCO*, 20:278.
12. Brunner, K. W., and Jungi, W. (1979): Mono- and combination chemotherapy with VP-16-213 in small-cell lung cancer (SLC). *Proc. Am. Assoc. Cancer Res. and ASCO*, 20:308.
13. Brunner, K. W., Sonntag, R. W., Ryssell, H. J., and Cavalli, F. (1976): Comparison of the biologic activity of VP-16 given i.v. and orally in capsules or drink ampules. *Cancer Treat. Rep.*, 60:1,377–1,379.
14. Cavalli, F., Hasler, E., Ryssell, H. J., Sonntag, R. W., and Brunner, K. W. (1977): A combination of cyclophosphamide, methotrexate, vincristine, and VP-16-213 (NSC-141540) in the treatment of bronchogenic carcinoma. *Tumori*, 63:169–173.
15. Cavalli, F., Klepp, O., Renard, J., Röhrt, M., and Alberto, P.: A phase II study of oral VP-16-213 in nonseminomatous testicular cancer. *Eur. J. Cancer (in press)*.
16. Cavalli, F., Ryssell, H. J., Batz, K., Sonntag, R. W., and Brunner, K. W. (1975): Erste Resultate mit dem Epipodophyllotoxin—Derivat VP-16-213 bei der Behand Lung akuter Leukämien. *Schweiz. Med. Wschr.*, 105:250–253.
17. Cavalli, F., Sonntag, R., and Brunner, K. W. (1975): Epipodopyllotoxin VP-16-213 in acute nonlymphoblastic leukaemia. *Br. Med. J.*, 1:227.
18. Cavalli, F., Sonntag, R. W., and Brunner, K. W. (1977): Epipodophyllin derivative (VP-16-213) in treatment of solid tumors. *Lancet*, 2:362.
19. Cavalli, F., Sonntag, R. W., Ryssell, H. J., and Brunner, K. W. (1977): Lack of severe hypotension with VP-16-213 administration directly i.v. *Cancer Treat. Rep.*, 61:1,411.
20. Cavalli, F., Sonntag, R. W., Jungi, F., Senn, H. J., and Brunner, K. W. (1978): VP-16-213 monochemotherapy for remission induction of small-cell lung cancer: A randomized trial using three dosage schedules. *Cancer Treat. Rep.*, 62:473–475.

21. Cecil, J. W., Quagliana, J. M., Coltman, C. A., Al-Sarraf, M., Thigpen, T., and Groope, C. W. (1978): Evaluation of VP-16-213 in malignant lymphoma and melanoma. *Cancer Treat. Rep.*, 62:801–803.

22. Chahinian, A. P., Chamberlin, K. B., and Holland, J. F. (1979): A new four-drug combination in advanced lung cancer (LC). *Proc. Am. Cancer Res. and ASCO*, 20:437.

23. Chakravorty, R. C., Sarkar, S. K., Sen, S., and Mukerji, B. (1967): Human anticancer effect of podophyllum derivatives (SPG and SPI). *Br. J. Cancer.*, 21:33–39.

24. Chard, R. L., Krivit, W., Bleyer, W. A., and Hammond, D. (1979): Phase II study of VP-16-213 in childhood malignant disease: A Children's Cancer Study Group Report. *Cancer Treat. Rep.*, 63:1,755–1,759.

25. Cohen, M. H., Broder, L. E., Fossieck, B. E., Ihde, D. C., and Minna, J. D. (1977): Phase II clinical trial of weekly administration of VP-16-213 in small-cell bronchogenic carcinoma. *Cancer Treat. Rep.*, 61:489–490.

26. Creaven, P. J., and Allen, L. M. (1975): E.P.E.G., a new antineoplastic epipodophyllotoxin. *Clin. Pharmacol. Ther.*, 18:221–226.

27. Creaven, P. J., and Allen, L. M. (1975): PTG, a new antineoplastic epipodophyllotoxin. *Clin. Pharmacol. Ther.*, 18:227–233.

28. Creaven, P. J., Newman, S. J., Selawry, O. S., Cohen, M. H., and Primack, A. (1974): Phase I clinical trial of weekly administration of 4'-demethylepipodophillotoxin-9-(4,6-O-ethylidene-β-D-glucopyranoside) NSC-141540: VP-16-213. *Cancer Chemother. Rep.*, 58:901–907

29. Dombernowsky, P., Hansen, H. H., Sorensen, S., and Østerlind, K. (1979): Sequential versus nonsequential combination chemotherapy using 6 drugs in advanced small-cell carcinoma (sm. a.c.). A comparative trial including 146 patients. *Proc. Am. Assoc. Cancer Res. and ASCO*, 20:277.

30. Dombernowsky, P., and Nissen, N. I. (1973): Schedule dependency of the antileukemic activity of the podophyllotoxin derivative VP-16-213 in L1210 leukemia. *Acta Pathol. Microbiol. Scand.*, 81:715–724.

31. Douglass, H. O., Jr., Lavin, P. T., Evans, J. T., Mittelman, A., and Carbone, P. P. (1979): Phase II evaluation of diglycoaldehyde, VP-16-213, and the combination of Methyl CCNU and β-2'-deoxythioguanosine in previously treated patients with colorectal cancer: An Eastern Cooperative Oncology Group study (EST-1275). *Cancer Treat. Rep.*, 63:1,355–1,357.

32. Drewinko, B., and Barlogie, B. (1976): Survival and cycle progression delay of human lymphoma cells *in vitro* exposed to VP-16-213. *Cancer Treat. Rep.*, 60:1,295–1,306.

33. Dubousky, D., Kernoff, L., and Jacobs, P. (1978): Rapid remission induction in adult acute nonlymphoblastic leukemia. *Eur. J. Cancer.*, 14:1,179–1,183.

34. Eagan, R. T., Ahmann, D. L., Hahn, R. G., and O'Connell, M. J. (1975): Pilot study to determine an intermittent dose schedule for VP-16-213. *Proc. Am. Assoc. Cancer Res. and ASCO*, 16:55.

35. Eagan, R. T., Carr, D. T., Frytak, S., Rubin, J., and Lee, R. E. (1976): VP-16-213 versus polychemotherapy in patients with advanced small-cell lung cancer. *Cancer Treat. Rep.*, 60:949–951.

36. Eagan, R. T., Ingle, J. N., Creagan, E. T., Frytak, S., Kvols, L. K., Rubin, J., and McMahon, R. T. (1978): VP-16-213 chemotherapy for advanced squamous cell carcinoma and adenocarcinoma of the lung. *Cancer Treat. Rep.*, 62:843–844.

37. Edmonson, J. H., Decker, D. G., Malkasian, G. D., Webb, M. J., and Jorgensen, E. O. (1978): Phase II evaluation of VP-16-213 (NSC-141540) in patients with advanced ovarian carcinoma resistant to alkylating agents. *Gynecol. Oncol.*. 6:7–9.

38. EORTC Clinical Screening Group (1973): Epipodophyllotoxin VP-16-213 in treatment of acute leukemias, haemosarcomas, and solid tumors. *Br. Med. J.*, 3:199–202.

39. Estapé, J., Millá, A., Agusti, A., Sanchez-Lloret, J., Palacin, A., and Soriano, E. (1979): VP-16-213 (VP-16) and cyclophosphamide in the treatment of primitive lung cancer in phase M_1. *Cancer*, 43:72–77.

40. Estapé, J., Millá, A., Agusti, A., Sanchez-Lloret, J., and Rozman, C. (1980): VP-16-213 plus cyclophosphamide in lung cancer. In *Abstracts of the EORTC Symposium on New Approaches in Cancer Therapy*, p. 2, Madrid, October 2–3

41. Falkson, G., and Synman, H. J. (1964): Experience with chemotherapy of cancer at the University of Pretoria. *Acta UICC.*, 20:439–446.

42. Falkson, G., Van Dyk, J. J., Van Eden, E. B., Van Der Merwe, A. M., Van Der Berg, J. A., and Falkson, H. C. (1975): A clinical trial of the oral form of 4'-demethylepipodophyllotoxin-β-D-ethylideneglucose (NS C-141540) VP-16-213. *Cancer*, 35:1,141–1,144.

43. Fontana, J. A. (1979): Radiation recall associated with VP-16-213 therapy. *Cancer Treat. Rep.*, 63:224–225.
44. Geran, R. I., Congleton, G. F., Dudeck, L. E., Abbott, B. J., and Gargus, J. L. (1974): A mouse ependymoblastoma as an experimental model for screening potential antineoplastic drugs. *Cancer Chemother. Rep.*, Part 2. 4:53–87.
45. Getaz, E. P., and Staples, W. G. (1977): Chronic myelomonocytic leukemia: A case report. *S. Afr. Med. J.*, 51:852–853.
46. Grieder, A., Maurer, R., and Stähelin, H. (1977): Comparative study of early effects of epipodophyllotoxin derivatives and other cytostatic agents on mastocytoma cultures. *Cancer Res.*, 37:2,998–3,005.
47. Hahn, R. G., Bauer, M., Wolter, J., Creech, R., Bennett, J. M., and Wampler, G. (1979): Phase II study of single agent therapy with megestrol acetate, VP-16-213, cyclophosphamide, and dianhydrogalactitol in advanced renal cell cancer. *Cancer Treat. Rep.*, 63:513–515.
48. Hansen, M., Hirsch, F., Dombernowsky, P., and Hansen, H. H. (1977): Treatment of small-cell anaplastic carcinoma of the lung with the oral solution of VP-16-213 (NSC-141540). *Cancer*, 40:633–637.
49. Hartwell, J. L. (1947): α-Peltatin, a new compound isolated from *Podophyllum peltatum*. *J. Am. Chem. Soc.*, 69:2,918–2,921.
50. Hartwell, J. L. (1976): Types of anticancer agents isolated from plants. *Cancer Treat. Rep.*, 60:1,031–1,067.
51. Horwitz, S. B., and Loike, J. O. (1977): A comparison of the mechanism of action of VP-16-213 and podophyllotoxin. *Lloydia*, 40:82–89.
52. Issell, B. F., and Crooke, S. T. (1979): Etoposide (VP-16-213). *Cancer Treat. Rev.*, 6:107–124.
53. Jacobs, P. (1976): VP-16-213 in the treatment of acute leukemia. *Cancer Treat. Rep.*, 60:967.
54. Jacobs, P., Dubowsky, D., Houggard, M., and Comay, S. (1975): Epipodophyllotoxin VP-16-213 in acute nonlymphoblastic leukaemia. *Br. Med. J.*, 1:396.
55. Jacobs, P., King, H., Cassidy, F., and Dent, D. (1979): The treatment of diffuse lymphocytic lymphoma (large-cell) with VP-16-213. *Proc. Am. Assoc. Cancer Res. and ASCO*, 20:280.
56. Jacobs, P., King, H. S., and Gordon, W. (1975): Chemotherapy of mycosis fungoides. *S. Afr. Med. J.*, 49:1,286.
57. Jacobs, P., King, H. S., and Sealy, G. R. H. (1975): Epipodophyllotoxin (VP-16-213) in the treatment of diffuse histiocytic lymphoma. *S. Afr. Med. J.*, 49:483–485.
58. Jungi, W. F., and Senn, H. J. (1975): Clinical study of the new podophyllotoxin derivative, 4'-demethylepipodophyllotoxin-9-(4,6-O-ethylidene-β-D-glucopyranoside) (NSC-141540; VP-16-213), in solid tumors in man. *Cancer Chemother. Rep.*, 59:737–742.
59. Kaplan, I. W. (1942): Condyloma acuminata. *New Orleans Med. Surg. J.*, 94:388–390.
60. Keller-Juslen, C., Kuhn, M., Von Wartburg, G., and Stähellin, H. (1971): Synthesis and antimitotic activity of glycosidic ligand derivatives related to podophyllotoxin. *J. Med. Chem.*, 14:936–940.
61. King, L., and Sullivan, M. (1946): Colchicine-like effect of podophyllotoxin. *Science*, 104:244–245.
62. Krishan, A., Paika, K., and Frei, E., III. (1975): Cytofluorometric studies on the action of podophyllotoxin and epipodophyllotoxins (VM-26, VP-16-213) on the cell cycle traverse of human lymphoblasts. *J. Cell Biol.*, 66:521–530.
63. Lau, M. E., Hansen, H. H., Nissen, N. I., and Pedersen, H. (1979): Phase I trial of a new form of an oral administration of VP-16-213. *Cancer Treat. Rep.*, 63:485–487.
64. Loike, J. D., Brewer, C. F., Sternlicht, H., Gensler, W. J., and Horwitz, S. B. (1978): Structure-activity study of the inhibition of microtubule assembly *in vitro* by podophyllotoxin and its congeners. *Cancer Res.*, 38:2,688–2,693.
65. Loike, J. D., and Horwitz, S. B. (1976a): Effects of VP-16-213 on microtubule assembly *in vitro* and nucleoside transport in HeLa cells. *Biochemistry.*, 15:5,435–5,442.
66. Loike, J. D., and Horwitz, S. B. (1976b): Effects of VP-16-213 on the intracellular degradation of DNA in HeLa cells. *Biochemistry.*, 15:5,443–5,448.
67. Mabel, J. A., and Little, A. D. (1979): Therapeutic synergism in murine tumors for combinations of cis-platinum with VP-16-213 or BCNU. *Proc. Am. Assoc. Cancer Res. and ASCO*, 230:929.
68. Mathe, G., Schwarzenberg, L., Pouillart, P., Oldham, R., Weiner, R., Jasmin, C., Rosenfeld, C., Hayat, M., Misset, J. L., Musset, M., Schneider, M., Amiel, J. L., and De Vassal, F. (1974): Two epipodophyllotoxin derivatives, VM-26 and VP-16-213, in the treatment of leukemias, hematosarcomas, and lymphomas. *Cancer*, 34:985–992.

69. Misra, N. C., and Roberts, D. (1975): Inhibition by 4'-demethylepipodophyllotoxin-9-(4,6-O-2-thenylidene-β-D-glucopyranoside) of human lymphoblast cultures in G2 phase of the cell cycle. *Cancer Res.*, 35:99–105.

70. Mosijczuk, A. D., Ruyman, F. B., Mease, A. D., and Bernier, R. D. (1979): Anthracycline cardiomyopathy in children. Report of two cases. *Cancer*, 44:1,582–1,587.

71. Muggia, F. M., Selawry, O. S., and Hansen, H. H. (1971): Clinical studies with a new podophyllotoxin derivative, epipodophyllotoxin, 4'-Demethyl-9-(4,6-O-2-thenylidene-β-D-glucopyranoside) (NSC-122819). *Cancer Chemother. Rep.*, 55:575–581.

72. Newlands, E. S., and Bagshawe, K. D. (1977): Epipodophyllotoxin derivative (VP-16-213) in malignant teratomas and choriocarcinomas. *Lancet*, 2:87.

73. Nissen, N. I., Dombernowsky, P., Hansen, H. H., and Larsen, V. (1976): Phase I clinical trial of an oral solution of VP-16-213. *Cancer Treat. Rep.*, 60:943–945.

74. Nissen, N. I., Hansen, H. H., Pedersen, H., Stryer, I., Dombernowsky, P., and Hessellund, M. (1975): Clinical trial of the oral form of a new podophyllotoxin derivative, VP-16-213 (NSC-141540) in patients with advanced neoplastic disease. *Cancer Chemother. Rep.*, 59:1,027–1,029.

75. Nissen, N. I., Larsen, V., Pedersen, H., and Thomson, K. (1972): Phase I clinical trials of a new antitumor agent: 4'-Demethylepipodophyllotoxin-9-(4,6-O-ethylidene-β-D-glucopyranoside), VP-16-213. *Cancer Chemother. Rep.*, 56:769–777.

76. Nissen, N. I., Pajak, T. F., Leone, L. A., Bloomfield, C. D., Kennedy, B. J., Ellison, R. R., Silver, R. T., Weiss, R. B., Cuttner, J., Falkson, G., Kung, F., Bergevin, P. R., and Holland, J. F. (1980): Clinical trial of VP-16-213 (NSC-141540) i.v. twice weekly in advanced neoplastic disease. A study by the Cancer and Leukemia Group B. *Cancer*, 45:232–235.

77. O'Connell, M. J., Silverstein, M. N., Kieley, J. M., and White, W. L. (1977): Pilot study of two adriamycin-based regimens in patients with advanced malignant lymphomas. *Cancer Treat. Rep.*, 61:65–68.

78. Odom, L. F., Rose, B., and Tubergen, D. G. (1979): A successful induction regimen for childhood acute nonlymphoblastic leukemia (ANLL). *Proc. Am. Assoc. Cancer Res. and ASCO*, 20:440.

79. Perry, M. C., Moertel, C. G., Schult, A. J., Reitemeier, R. J., Hahn, R. G., and Hahn, G. (1976): Phase II studies of dianhydrogalactitol and VP-16-213 in colorectal cancer. *Cancer Treat. Rep.*, 60:1,247–1,250.

80. Pethema. Spanish Cooperative Group. Protocolo para el diagnóstico y tratamiento de los linfomas no Hodgkin, estadios III y IV. Protocol X/80.

81. Radice, P. A., Bunn, P. A., and Ihde, D. C. (1979): Therapeutic trials with VP-16-213 and VM-26. Active agents in small cell lung cancer, non-Hodgkin's lymphomas, and other malignancies. *Cancer Treat. Rep.*, 63:1,231–1,239.

82. Rivera, G., Avery, T., and Pratt, C. (1975): 4'-Demethylepipodophyllotoxin-9-(4,6-O-2-thenylidene-β-D-glucopyranoside) (VM-26) and 4'-demethylepipodophyllotoxin-9-(4,6-O-ethylidene-β-D-glucopyranoside) (VP-16-213) in childhood cancer: Preliminary observations. *Cancer Chemother. Rep.*, 59:743–749.

83. Rivera, G., Avery, T., and Roberts, D. (1975): Response of L1210 to combinations of cytosine arabinoside and VM-26 or VP-16-213. *Eur. J. Cancer*, 11:639–647.

84. Rozencweig, M., Von Hoff, D., Henney, J. H., and Muggia, F. M. (1977): VM-26 and VP-16-213: A comparative analysis. *Cancer*, 40:334–342.

85. Ryssel, H. J., Hasler, E., Sonntag, G. W., Cavalli, F., Martin, J., Tschopp, L., and Brunner, K. W. (1977): VP-16-213 in kombination mit Endoxan, Methotrexat, und Oncovin als polychemotherapic beim bronchuskartinom. *Schweiz, Med. Wschr.*, 107:912–915.

86. Schabel, F. M., Trader, M. W., Laster, W. R., Jr., Corbett, T. A., and Griswold, D. P., Jr. (1979): Cis-dichlorodiammineplatinum. II. Combination chemotherapy and cross-resistence studies with tumors of mice. *Cancer Treat. Rep.*, 63:1,459–1,473.

87. Schecter, J. P., and Jones, S. E. (1975): Myocardial infarction in a 27-year-old woman: Possible complication of treatment with VP-16-213 (NSC-141540), mediastinal irradiation, or both (Letter). *Cancer Treat. Rep.*, 59:887.

88. Schmieder, H. A., Jungi, W. F., Mayr, A. C., and Senn, H. J. (1979): Erfahrungen mit VP-16 in kombination mit Cyclophosphamid oder Adriamycin beim anaplastischem, vorwiegend Kleinzelligen Bronchuskarzinom. *Schweiz. Med. Wschr.*, 109:841–844.

89. Sierocki, J. S., Hilaris, B. S., Hopfan, S., Martini, N., Barton, D., Golbey, R. B., and Wittes, R. E. (1979): Cis-dichlorodiammineplatinum (II) and VP-16-213: An active induction regimen for small cell carcinoma of the lung. *Cancer Treat. Rep.*, 63:1,593–1,597.

90. Slayton, R. E., Creasman, W. T., Petty, W., Bundy, B., and Blessing, J. A. (1979): Phase II trial of VP-16-213 in the treatment of advanced squamous cell carcinoma of the cervix and adenocarcinoma of the ovary: A Gynecologic-Oncology Group Study. *Cancer Treat, Rep.*, 63:2,089–2,092.

91. Smith, I. E., Gerken, M. W., Clink, H. M., and McElwain, T. J. (1976): VP-16-213 in acute myelogenous leukemia. *Postgrad. Med.*, 52:66–70.

92. Stähelin, H. (1973): Activity of a new glycosidic ligand derivative (VP-16-213) related to podophyllotoxin in experimental tumors. *Eur. J. Cancer*, 9:215–221.

93. Tucker, R. D., Ferguson, A., Van Wyk, C., Sealy, R., Hewitson, R., and Levin, R. (1978): Chemotherapy of small-cell carcinoma of the lung with VP-16-213. *Cancer*, 41:1,710–1,714.

94. Vaitkevicius, V. K., and Reed, H. L. (1966): Clinical studies with podophyllum compounds SPI-77 (NSC-72274) and SPG-827 (NSC-42076). *Cancer Chemother. Rep.*, 50:565–571.

95. Van Echo, D. A., Aisner, J., Wiernik, P. H., Morris, D., and Serpik, A. (1979): Combination chemotherapy of advanced breast cancer with adriamycin and VP-16-213. *Proc. Am. Assoc. Cancer Rep. and ASCO*, 228:921.

96. Van Echo, D. A., Lichtenfeld, K. M., and Wiernik, P. H. (1977): Vinblastine, 5-azacytidine, and VP-16-213 therapy for previously treated patients with acute nonlymphocytic leukemia. *Cancer Treat. Rep.*, 61:1,599–1,602.

97. Vietti, T. J., Valeriote, F. A., Kalish, R., and Coulter, D. (1978): Kinetics of cytotoxicity of VM-26 and VP-16-213 on L1212 leukemia and hematopoietic stem cells. *Cancer Treat. Rep.*, 62:1,313–1,320.

98. Vincent, R. G., Wilson, H. E., Lane, W. W., Chen, T. Y., Raza, S., Gutierrez, A., and Caracandas, J. E. (1981): Progress in the chemotherapy of small-cell carcinoma of the lung. *Cancer*, 47:229–235.

99. Wang, J. J., and Chervinsky, D. S. (1978): Effect of podophyllotoxin derivative (VP-16-213) on nucleic acid and protein biosynthesis in L1212 leukemic cells. *Proc. Am. Assoc. Cancer Rep. and ASCO*, 14:100.

100. Williams, S. D., Einhorn, L. H., Greco, F. A., Oldham, R., and Fletcher, R. (1980): VP-16-213 salvage therapy for refractory germinal neoplasms. *Cancer*, 46:2,154–2,158.

101. Young, C. W., Ihde, D. C., and Von Stubbe, W. (1973): Preliminary clinical trial of 4′-demethylepipodophyllotoxin-β-D-ethylideneglucoside (VP-16-213). *Proc. Am. Assoc. Cancer Res.*, 14:60.

New Approaches in Cancer Therapy,
edited by H. Cortés Funes and M. Rozencweig.
Raven Press, New York © 1982.

Phase II–III Evaluation of Cisplatin

A. Moyano and H. Cortés Funes

Seccion de Oncologia Medica, Ciudad Sanitaria de la Seguridad Social
"1º de Octubre," Madrid 17, Spain

In 1965 Rosenberg et al. (27) suggested that platinum compounds were potentially valuable chemotherapeutic agents. Cisplatin (DDP) was first used in phase I clinical trials in 1969, and responses in testicular cancer, bladder cancer, prostatic cancer, ovarian cancer, head and neck cancer, and lymphomas were observed (2–5,7–13,22,28,29,31,34,36). Some success has been observed in treating childhood malignancies (1,6,14,24,25,33).

The mechanism of action of DDP has been widely discussed elsewhere; the drug essentially produces selective inhibition of deoxyribonucleic acid (DNA) synthesis. Chloride ligands of DDP possibly act as leaving groups, permitting alkylation of the nucleophilic moieties of DNA; intra- and interstrand cross-linking of DNA have been reported (15,26). Other mechanisms of action have also been suggested (15).

Numerous investigators (17,18) have shown that nephrotoxicity is the main limitation of DDP use. However, this can be circumvented with adequate hydration before and after treatment (16,30). Other toxicities, such as ototoxicity, neurotoxicity, gastrointestinal toxicity, hepatotoxicity, and myelosuppression have been shown to be less severe (20,21,23).

One of the potentially desirable characteristics of DDP is its synergistic effect with other chemotherapeutic agents such as cyclophosphamide, adriamycin, and VP-16-213 (25).

Since September of 1976, DDP has been investigated at the Seccion de Oncologia Medica of Hospital "1° de Octubre" in Madrid in various phase II and III programs, coordinated by the Cancer Therapy Evaluation Program of the Nutritional Cancer Institute (USA). This chapter details the results of these clinical trials.

MATERIALS AND METHODS

All patients in this study received treatment with DDP either as a single agent or as part of a combination regimen. Most patients had advanced disease resistant to standard chemotherapy.

Dr. Moyano's present address is Baltimore Cancer Research Program, NCI, DCT, University of Maryland at Baltimore, Baltimore, Maryland 21201.

Prior to DDP treatment, prehydration using 3,000 cc of dextrose 5 normal saline (D5NS) plus 60 mEq of KCl was given for 12 hr. Then, 25 g of mannitol were injected as a rapid infusion and DDP was given as a 1-hr infusion. Another 25 g of mannitol and 2,500 to 3,000 cc of D5NS plus 40 mEq of KCl were given over the next 12 hr to complete the hydration. Support therapy for nausea and vomiting was given prior to treatment and as needed. The first 48 hr after treatment, an oral supplement of magnesium was added to prevent hypomagnesemia.

Conventional criteria for response were used (WHO). Complete remission (CR) was defined as disappearance of all measurable disease for a minimum of 1 month and partial remission (PR) was defined as a reduction of measurable disease by more than 50%.

PATIENT CHARACTERISTICS

Two hundred and twenty-seven patients were treated in this study. Twenty-one patients received DDP as a single agent and 206 received it in combination (Table 1). In the first group, 15 patients were males and 6 were females. The median age was 28.5 years and the median follow-up time was 6.3 months. In the second group, 169 patients were males and 37 were females. The median age was 38 years and the median follow-up time was 9.4 months.

RESULTS

Receiving DDP as a single agent, only 4 of 21 patients achieved PR (19%). These patients had neuroblastoma, Ewing sarcoma, gastric cancer, and bladder carcinoma (Table 2).

DDP was given in combination with other chemotherapeutic agents as shown in Table 3. These included:

1. DDP plus vinblastine and bleomycin for testicular tumors in two different regimens.
2. DDP plus cyclophosphamide and VP-16 for small-cell carcinoma of the lung.
3. DDP plus cyclophosphamide and adriamycin for non-small-cell lung cancer.
4. DDP plus bleomycin for head and neck carcinoma.
5. DDP plus cyclophosphamide for osteogenic sarcoma.
6. DDP plus cyclophosphamide and adriamycin for a group of patients with miscellaneous malignancies.

These groups of patients will be analyzed separately.

Results by Tumor Type

Germ Cell Tumors

Fifty-six patients with advanced germ cell tumors underwent treatment with two different combinations of DDP, vinblastine and bleomycin. They were classified in two different groups according to the treatment regimen. Nineteen patients treated

TABLE 1. *DDP (phase II and III)*

Patient characteristics	Alone	In combination	Total
Total number	21	206	227
Sex			
Male	15	169	184
Female	6	37	43
Age (year)			
Median	28.5	38	33.2
Range	(4–53)	(2–69)	(2–69)
Follow-up (month)			
Median	6.3	9.4	7.8
Range	(2–9)	(2–45+)	(2–45+)
Cycles (no.)	105	1,088	1,193
Median/patient	3.2	5.3	4.2

TABLE 2. *Single agent activity of DDP*

Tumor	No. of patients	PR	CR
Synoviosarcoma	1	—	—
Rhabdomyosarcoma	2	—	—
Esophagus cancer	1	—	—
Neuroblastoma	2	1	—
Ewing sarcoma	2	1	—
Breast cancer	2	—	—
Gastric cancer	1	1	—
Non-Hodgkin lymphoma	1	—	—
Hodgkin disease	1	—	—
Melanoma	3	—	—
Thyroid cancer	2	—	—
Bladder cancer	3	1	—
Total	21	4 (19%)	

with the first regimen described in Table 3 achieved CR (37.5%) and, of these, 6 remain free of disease with a median follow-up of 14.3 months (2 to 45+). Thirty-seven patients received the second regimen. Twenty-eight patients achieved CR (75.6%). Twenty-five patients remain in CR with a median follow-up of 9.7 months (1 to 19+) (Table 4). Two patients developed recurrence and another died of pulmonary embolism 3 months after CR was achieved.

Lung Carcinoma

Twenty-four patients with small-cell lung carcinoma were treated. Fourteen presented with extensive disease and 10 with limited disease. Of 14 patients with extensive disease, 2 achieved CR and 3 achieved PR. Among 10 patients with

TABLE 3. *DDP in combination*

		Doses[a]					
Tumor	No. of patients	DDP (mg/m²)	VLB (mg/m²)	BLM (U)	CTX (mg/m²)	ADM (mg/m²)	VP-16 (mg/m²)
Germ cell tumors	56	20 × 5	3 × 2	30 × 12[b]	—	—	—
(Phase I: 19)		100	6 × 2	30 × 5[c]	—	—	—
(Phase II: 37)							
Lung cancer							
Small cell	24	60	—	—	800	—	120
Other than small cell	37	80	—	—	600	40	—
Head and neck	47	120	—	30 × 5[c]	—	—	—
Osteogenic sarcoma	29	60	—	—	600	—	—
Miscellaneous	13	80	—	—	600	40	—
Total	206						

[a]VLB = vinblastine; BLM = bleomycin; CTX = cyclophosphamide; ADM = adriamycin; VP-16 = epipodophylotoxin.
[b]Given i.v. push weekly.
[c]Given in continuous infusion.

TABLE 4. *Results of treatment with DDP in combination*

Combination for (tumor)		Patients (no.)	Overall responses	CR
DDP-DLM-VLB	1st group	19	19 (100%)	7 (37%)
(germ cell tumors)	2nd group	37	34 (91.8%)	28 (75.6%)
DDP-VP-16-CTX		24	14 (58.3%)	6 (25%)
(small cell lung cancer)				
DDP-ADM-CTX		37	15 (40.5%)	0 —
(non-small cell)				
DDP-BLM		21	10 (47.6%)	1
(metastatic or relapsed head and neck and previously treated)				
DDP-BLM		26	17 (65.3%)	2
(head and neck without prior treatment)				
DDP-CTX		11	5 (45.4%)	—
(metastatic osteogenic sarcoma)				
DDP-CTX		18	(9/18 developed metastasis in 7.8 months)	
(metastatic osteogenic sarcoma)				
DDP-ADM-CTX		13	5 (38.4%)	—
(miscellaneous)				
Total		206	117	

limited disease, there were 4 CR and 5 PR. The median survival was 7.5 months in patients with limited disease and 5.1 months in patients with extensive disease. When both groups were analyzed together, 14 patients responded (58.3%) and 6 patients achieved CR (25%). Thirty-seven patients with non-small-cell lung carcinoma were treated. Only 15 patients (40.5%) achieved PR. No one achieved CR. All patients had extensive disease at the time of the treatment. The median performance status was 2. Median survival was 6.9 months. No significant difference in response and survival was found when the different histological categories were compared (squamous carcinoma 42%, 8.7 months; adenocarcinoma 36%, 8.9 months; and giant-cell carcinoma 42%, 7.9 months) (Table 4).

Head and Neck Tumors

Forty-seven patients with head and neck primary tumors were treated. Twenty-one had local recurrence, distant metastases, or both at the time of the treatment, and all of these patients were previously treated. Of these 21 patients, only 10 (47.6%) responded and 1 had CR. The median time of response was 7.9 months.

Twenty-six patients presented with locally advanced disease. The majority of these patients had poor prognostic factors, such as weight loss in the last month and low nutritional status. Median performance status was 2. None of these patients had received previous treatment. They were treated with two courses of chemotherapy followed by radiotherapy. Evaluation before the radiation treatment showed that 17 responded (65.3%) and 2 of these achieved CR. Among the 15 patients with PR, 7 achieved CR after radiation therapy.

Osteogenic Sarcoma

Twenty-nine patients with osteogenic sarcoma were treated. Eleven patients presented with lung metastases, and 5 of them (45.5%) achieved PR.

Eighteen patients received a DDP regimen as adjuvant therapy after radical surgery. Operation consisted of amputation at the nearest articulation above the tumor in 27 cases and disarticulation in 2 cases. Nine patients developed metastases within a median time of 7.8 months (Table 4).

Miscellaneous

Four patients with ovarian carcinoma, 3 patients with bladder carcinoma, 4 with carcinoma of unknown origin, 1 with renal carcinoma, and 1 with neuroblastoma were treated. Five patients (38.4%) achieved PR. These responses occurred in 2 patients with bladder carcinoma and 3 with ovarian carcinoma.

TOXICITY

Table 5 shows the side effects of DDP given alone or in combination. Nausea and vomiting were reported in 100% of the patients. These symptoms began 1 hr after DDP was administered and they lasted 2 to 24 hr. Chlorpropamide and chlorpromazine could not control them. Recently we used a haloperidol derivative (Droperidol) with some preliminary successful results. Renal toxicity was seen in less than 10% of treated patients. Only 2 patients developed irreversible renal failure. The remaining patients recovered from nephrotoxicity when the treatment was discontinued. We studied the changes of renal function measuring blood urea nitrogen (BUN), creatinine, and creatinine clearance in patients with germ cell tumors

TABLE 5. *DDP toxicity (phase II and III)*

Side effects	Single agent	In combination[a]					Total
Protocol		A	B	C	D	E	
No. of patients	21	56	61	47	29	13	227
Gastrointestinal							
Nausea, vomiting	21	56	61	47	29	13	227 (100%)
Renal							
Serum creatinine $\geq$ 2 mg%	4	7	3	4	—	2	20 (8.8%)
Creatinine clearance $\leq$ 50 ml/m	4	8	5	3	—	2	22 (9.6%)
Irreversible renal failure	—	1	—	1	—	—	2 (0.8%)
Neurological[b]							
Tinnitus	2	7	1	3	—	—	13 (5.7%)
Paresthesias–tendon reflexes	—	10/10	8/8	5/5	2/2	—	25/25 (100%)
EMG disturbances	—	10/10	8/8	5/5	2/2	—	25/25 (100%)
Hepatic	—	—	1	1	—	—	2 (0.8%)
Allergies	—	—	—	—	2	—	2 (0.8%)
Hematological							
WBC $\leq$ 2,000/mm^3	1	32	15	7	2	1	58 (25.5%)
PTS $\leq$ 100,000/mm^3		19	8	4	—	1	32 (14%)

[a]A: germ cell tumors; B: lung cancer; C: head and neck cancer; D: osteogenic sarcoma; and E: miscellaneous.
[b]Neurological toxicity studies were done only in 25 patients.

since these patients were long-term survivors and received large total cumulative doses of DDP. We correlated renal function and the total dose received at 3, 6, 12, and 18 months. Patients given total doses between 1,000 and 1,500 mg DDP did not experience severe renal toxicity and there was a tendency to recover from renal function abnormalities after treatment withdrawal (23).

Peripheral neurotoxicity was the main neurological toxicity associated with DDP. It presented as paresthesias, decrease in peripheral reflexes, and motor weakness. Twenty patients who had total cumulative doses of DDP over 500 mg were studied for peripheral neuropathy. These 20 patients showed paresthesias, decrease of reflexes, and electromyogram (EMG) alteration. In 2 of these patients, a nerve biopsy was done. Microscopic study showed axonal degeneration and demyelination. Ultrastructural studies showed condensation of the neurofilaments in the axons and vesiculization in Schwann cells and pericytes (21).

One patient died of toxic liver necrosis secondary to DDP. Other causes were excluded by autopsy which showed massive hepatic necrosis compatible with acute diffuse toxic necrosis.

Another patient with liver function test changes showed partial hepatic improvement after DDP was discontinued, but liver abnormalities persisted. Only 2 patients developed allergic reactions to DDP with facial edema, skin rash, and pruritus. When DDP was given as a single agent, only 1 patient developed transitory myelosuppression with white blood cell count (WBC) below 2,000/mm^3.

DISCUSSION

In our patients, when DDP was given as a single agent, response rate was relatively low. However, these patients had advanced stage of disease and had been previously treated. When the patients are considered according to specific tumor type, there are too few patients in each disease category to make any meaningful assessment of the antitumor activity.

Patients with germ cell tumors were treated with two different regimens using the same agents. In the first schedule, DDP was given at 20 mg/m^2 daily for 5 days. This regimen prolonged the hospitalization time without any apparent additional benefit. In the second regimen, the total dose of DDP was given in 1 day. The vinblastine dose was increased as reported by other authors (10,11). The CR rate for the second regimen was greater than the first ($p < 0.002$). Germ cell tumors from the ovary and mediastinum responded in the same way as primary testicular tumors. Seminoma is another particular type of tumor that, in our series, appeared to be very sensitive to this chemotherapy regimen (8).

Patients with small-cell lung carcinoma did not obtain as good results as those reported by others (2). This may substantiate the relatively minor role that DDP plays in the treatment of this disease (9). The short survival rate in the other histological types of lung cancer is another point to be emphasized. The use of DDP for lung tumors needs to be reconsidered.

DDP in head and neck tumors appears to be promising and may achieve higher activity than methotrexate. Considering the therapeutic results obtained in our and other series (13,19,35), DDP in combination with bleomycin may eventually be utilized as a standard chemotherapy treatment for previously untreated head and neck cancer patients.

Three of 5 patients with advanced osteogenic carcinoma responded when DDP was given together with cyclophosphamide. These preliminary results suggested that this combination may have some antitumor activity and prompted us to use the combination as adjuvant therapy after radical surgery. However, 50% of patients relapsed in 7.8 months. This would imply that this combination is probably not as effective as other established combinations. Further studies may be warranted to determine more accurately its activity in advanced disease.

Among the 13 patients classified in the miscellaneous group, 5 patients had responses. However, these occurred primarily in patients with ovarian and bladder carcinoma, and the combination of DDP, adriamycin, and cyclophosphamide has been shown by others (32,34) to be highly effective in ovarian carcinoma. The small number of patients with bladder cancer precludes any firm conclusion about the level of activity of this combination.

In conclusion, these studies have clearly shown that DDP is a highly effective antineoplastic agent with a wide spectrum of antitumor activity. These preliminary studies confirm the therapeutic role of DDP in head and neck cancer, testicular cancer, and ovarian cancer. The encouraging single agent activity of DDP has resulted in its incorporation into a variety of combination chemotherapy regimens in a number of tumor types. In most of these, a superiority of the combination over single agents remains to be demonstrated.

ACKNOWLEDGMENTS

We are indebted to Dr. Joseph Aisner for his critical evaluation of this chapter and Ms. McNamara and Ms. McWilliams for their technical help.

REFERENCES

1. Baum, E. S., Gaynon, L., Greenberg, L., Krivit, W., and Hammond, D. (1979): Cis-diamminechloroplatinum phase II study in osteogenic sarcoma of childhood: A report from Children's Cancer Study Group. *Cancer Treat. Rep.*, 63:1,621–1,629.
2. Cavalli, F., Jungi, W., Sontag, R. W., Nissen, N. I., and Holland, J. F. (1979): Phase II trials of cis-diamminedichloroplatinum (II) in advanced malignant lymphomas and small cell lung carcinoma: Preliminary results. *Cancer Treat. Rep.*, 63:1,599–1,603.
3. Cortes Funes, H. (1978): Cis-diamminedichloroplatinum (DDP), nuevo potente agente antiblastico. *Oncologia 80*, 1:18–23.
4. Cortes Funes, H., Alonso, E., Mendiola, C., Manas, A., Hernandez, V., and Moyano, A. (1981): Treatment of advanced non-small cell lung carcinoma with a combination of cyclophosphamide, adriamycin, and cis-platinum (CAP). *Cancer Clin. Trials (in press)*.
5. Cortes Funes, H., Moyano, A., Borovia, V., Valentin, V., Vicente, J., and Baena, L. (1978): Treatment of advanced germinal cell tumors nonseminomas with cis-diamminedichloroplatinum, bleomycin, and vinblastine. *Proceedings of the XII International Cancer Congress*, Buenos Aires. 3:119.
6. Cortes Funes, H., Moyano, A., and Manas, A. (1978): Cis-platinum (DDP) in combination with cyclophosphamide (CTX) for the treatment of metastatic osteogenic sarcoma. *IV Annual Meeting of the European Society of Medical Oncology*, Nice. 22:6.
7. Cortes Funes, H., Moyano, A., Manas, A., Ramos, A., Quiben, R., and Mendiola, C. (1980): Tratamiento de los tumores de celulas germinales avanzados con cis-platino, bleomicina, y vinblastina. *Oncologia 80*, 1:29–36.
8. Cortes Funes, H., Moyano, A., and Mendiola, C. (1981): Quimioterapia de los tumores de celulas germinales avanzados. *Oncologia 80 (in press)*.
9. Cortes Funes, H., Moyano, A., Ramos, A., Mendiola, C., Alonso, E., and Manas, A. (1981): Cis-platinum, cyclophosphamide, and VP-16 for the treatment of small-cell lung carcinoma. *Cancer Clin. Trials (in press)*.
10. Einhorn, L. (1978): Combination chemotherapy of disseminated testicular cancer with cis-diamminedichloroplatinum, vinblastine, and bleomycin (PVB). An update. *Proc. Am. Soc. Clin. Oncol. (Abstract)*, C-6:308.
11. Einhorn, L. (1979): Combination chemotherapy with cis-diamminedichloroplatinum (II) in disseminated testicular cancer. *Cancer Treat. Rep.*, 63:1,659–1,662.
12. Einhorn, L., and Donohue, J. (1977): Cis-diamminodichloroplatinum, vinblastine, and bleomycin as combination chemotherapy in disseminated testicular cancer. *Ann. Intern. Med.*, 87:293–295.
13. Elias, E. G., Chretien, P. B., and Monnard, E. (1979): Chemotherapy prior to local therapy in advanced squamous cell carcinoma of the head and neck. *Cancer*, 43:1,025–1,031.
14. Freeman, A. I., Ettinger, L. J., and Brecher, M. L. (1979): Cis-diamminedichloroplatinum (II) in childhood cancer. *Cancer Treat. Rep.*, 63:1,615–1,620.
15. Harder, H. C., and Rosenberg, B. (1970): Inhibitory effects of antitumor platinum compounds on DNA, RNA, and protein synthesis in mammalian cells *in vitro*. *Int. J. Cancer*, 6:207–216.
16. Hayes, D. M., Cvitkovic, E., Golbey, R., Scheiner, E., Helson, L., and Krakof, F. (1977): High dose cis-platinum diamminedichloride. Amelioration of renal toxicity by mannitol-induced diuresis. *Cancer*, 39:1,372–1,375.

17. Higby, D. J., Wallace, H. J., Jr., and Albert, D. (1974): Diamminedichloroplatinum in the chemotherapy of testicular tumors. *J. Urol.*, 112:100–105.
18. Hill, J. M., Loeb, E., and MacLellan, A. (1975): Clinical studies of platinum coordination compounds in the treatment of various malignant diseases. *Cancer Chemother. Rep.*, 59:647–659.
19. Hong, W. K., Shapshay, S. M., and Bhutani, R. (1979): Induction chemotherapy in advanced squamous head and neck carcinoma with high-dose cis-platinum and bleomycin infusion. *Cancer*, 44:19–25.
20. Kedar, A., Cohen, M. E., and Freeman, A. I. (1978): Peripheral neuropathy as a complication of cis-dichlorodiammineplatinum (II) treatment: A case report. *Cancer Treat. Rep.*, 62:819–821.
21. Manas, A., Cubillo, E., and Alonso, E. (1979): Monitoring peripheral neurotoxicity from cis-platinum (DDP). *V Annual Meeting of European Society of Medical Oncology*, Nice. 124:31.
22. Merrin, C. E. (1979): Treatment of genitourinary tumors with cis-diamminedichloroplatinum (II): Experience in 250 patients. *Cancer Treat. Rep.*, 63:1,579–1,584.
23. Moyano, A., Manas, A., Ramos, A., Mendiola, C., Usera, G., and Cortes Funes, H. (1979): Renal toxicity to different cumulative doses of cis-platinum (DDP). *V Annual Meeting of European Society of Medical Oncology*, Nice. 140:35.
24. Nitschke, R., Starling, K. A., Vats, T., and Bryan, H. (1978): Cis-diamminedichloroplatinum (NSC-119875) in childhood malignancies: A Southwest Oncology Group Study. *Med. Pediatr. Oncol.*, 4:127–130.
25. Ochs, J. J., Freeman, A. I., Douglas, H. O., Higby, D. S., Mindel, R., and Sinks, L. F. (1978): Cis-diamminedichloroplatinum (II) in advanced osteogenic sarcoma. *Cancer Treat. Rep.*, 62:239–245.
26. Page, R. H., Talley, R. W., and Buhagiar, J. (1977): The enhanced antitumor activity of cis-diamminedichloroplatinum (II) against murine tumors when combined with other agents. *J. Clin. Intern. Oncol.*, 7:96–104.
27. Rosenberg, B., van Camp, L., and Krigas, T. (1965): Inhibition of cell division in *Escherichia coli* by electrolysis products from a platinum electrode. *Nature*, 205:698–699.
28. Rossof, A. H., Bearden, J. D., III, and Coltman, C. A., Jr. (1976): Phase II evaluation of cis-diamminedichloroplatinum in lung cancer. *Cancer Treat. Rep.*, 60:1,679–1,681.
29. Rossof, A., Coltman, C., Jones, S., and Talley, W. (1979): Phase II evaluation of cis-dichlorodiammine platinum (II) in lymphomas: A Southwest Oncology Group Study. *Cancer Treat. Rep.*, 63:1,605–1,608.
30. Salem, P., Hall, S. W., Benjamin, R., Murphy, W., Taylor, J., and Bodey, G. (1978): Clinical phase I–II study of cis-dichlorodiammineplatinum (II) given by continuous I.V. infusion. *Cancer Treat. Rep.*, 62:1,553–1,555.
31. Samson, M. K., Stephens, R. L., and Rivkin, S. (1979): Vinblastine, bleomycin, and cis-dichlorodiammineplatinum (II) in disseminated testicular cancer. Preliminary report of a Southwest Oncology Group Study. *Cancer Treat. Rep.*, 63:1,663–1,667.
32. Thigpen, T., Shingleton, H., and Homesley, H. (1979): Cis-dichlorodiammineplatinum (II) in the treatment of gynecologic malignancies: Phase II trials by the Gynecologic Oncology Group. *Cancer Treat. Rep.*, 63:1,549–1,555.
33. Vietti, T. J., Nitschke, R., Starling, K. A., and Van Eys, J. (1979): Evaluation of cis-dichlorodiammineplatinum (II) in children with advanced malignant disease: Southwest Oncology Group Studies. *Cancer Treat. Rep.*, 63:1,611–1,614.
34. Wiltshaw, E., and Kroner, T. (1975): Phase II study of cis-dichlorodiammineplatinum (II) (NSC-119875) in advanced adenocarcinoma of the ovary. *Cancer Treat. Rev.*, 60:55–60.
35. Wittes, R. E., Cvitkovic, E., Shah, J., Gerald, F., and Strong, E. (1977): Cis-diamminedichloroplatinum (II) in the treatment of epidermoid carcinoma of the head and neck. *Cancer Treat. Rep.*, 61:359–361.
36. Yagoda, A. (1979): Phase II trials with cis-diamminechloroplatinum (II) in the treatment of urothelial cancer. *Cancer Treat. Rep.*, 63:1,565–1,572.

New Approaches in Cancer Therapy,
edited by H. Cortés Funes and M. Rozencweig.
Raven Press, New York © 1982.

Phase I Study of 4'-(9-Acridinylamino)-methanesulfon-*m*-anisidide in Children with Cancer

Gaston Rivera, Gary V. Dahl, and Charles B. Pratt

St. Jude Children's Research Hospital, Memphis, Tennessee 38101

4'-(9-Acridinylamino)-methanesulfon-*m*-anisidide (AMSA) (NSC-249992), an acridine derivative, is a potent new cytotoxic agent. AMSA was synthesized by Cain and Atwell and is thought to intercalate between nucleotide molecules (1,2). Currently, this compound is undergoing phase I and II clinical evaluations in the programs of the Investigational Drug Branch of the National Cancer Institute, Bethesda, Maryland. The study we present in this chapter is a phase I clinical trial performed exclusively in pediatric patients.

MATERIALS AND METHODS

Forty-one patients with a median age of 13 years (range, 3 to 21 years), whose diseases were refractory to conventional therapy, were studied. Twenty-four children had leukemia and 17 had solid tumors. Diagnoses included acute lymphoblastic leukemia (ALL) (13 patients), acute nonlymphoblastic leukemia (ANLL) (11 patients), osteosarcoma (7 patients), rhabdomyosarcoma (4 patients), malignant fibrous histiocytoma (2 patients), germ cell tumors (2 patients), synovial sarcoma (1 patient), and lymphoepithelioma (1 patient). Upon patients' admission to the study, evidence of normal renal and liver functions defined as serum creatinine and serum bilirubin <1.5 mg/dl and written informed consent of the patients' parents were required.

AMSA was provided by the National Cancer Institute and was formulated as two sterile liquids that were combined immediately prior to use. Each 2-ml flint ampul contained 1.5 ml of a 50-mg/ml solution of AMSA in anhydrous *N,N*-dimethylacetamide. Each 20-ml amber vial contained 13.5 ml of 0.0353 M lactic acid diluent. The solution was prepared by aseptically adding 1.5 ml of AMSA (50 mg/ml) to 13.5 ml of the diluent resulting in an orange-red solution containing 5 mg of the drug per ml. The drug was diluted in 100 ml of 5% dextrose in water due to the

---

Parts of this chapter were previously published in *Cancer Research*, 40:4250–4253, 1980, and are reprinted with permission of the publisher.

occurrence of phlebitis at higher concentrations. The schedule investigated was daily for 5 days every 2 to 3 weeks with a starting dosage of 1.3 mg/m^2/day. Treatments were given by slow i.v. injection over 10 to 20 min. In children with leukemia, dosages were escalated from 1.3 to 5.0, 30, 40, 100, 125, and 150 mg/m^2/day; in patients with solid tumors, dosages were escalated from 5.0 to 10, 15, 20, 25, and 50 mg/m^2/day. No patients were treated at more than one dosage level. Following the determination that there was no limiting toxicity at a given dosage, the next dosage level was investigated. Altogether, 74 courses of AMSA were administered.

Leukopenia and thrombocytopenia were defined as <3,000 leukocytes/mm^3 and <100,000 platelets/mm^3, respectively. An M-1 marrow was a cellular marrow with <5% blasts and no identifiable leukemia cells; an M-2 marrow contained 5 to 25% leukemic blasts; and an M-3 marrow contained >25% leukemic blasts.

RESULTS

Leukemia Patients

Forty-four courses of AMSA at seven different dosage levels were administered to the 24 patients with leukemia (Table 1). Toxicity was not encountered until the dosage level of 125 mg/m^2/day was reached. With both 125 and 150 mg/m^2/day, stomatitis, gastrointestinal toxicity, phlebitis, and alopecia were observed. Of the 6 patients treated with 125 mg/m^2/day for 5 days, 2 patients developed stomatitis; 4 patients developed gastrointestinal toxicity (3, vomiting; 1, diarrhea); 2 patients had phlebitis; and 1 patient developed alopecia. Of the 7 patients who received 150 mg/m^2/day for 5 days, 4 patients had vomiting related to chemotherapy; 2 patients had severe stomatitis; 2 patients had phlebitis; and 1 patient had alopecia. Hematopoietic toxicity could not be assessed in these patients due to advanced leukemia and previous multiple-agent chemotherapeutic treatments; however, at this dosage level, marrow recovery did not occur before 21 to 28 days.

Antileukemic activity was first evident at dosages of 30 mg/m^2/day and was seen at each subsequent higher dosage. At 30 to 40 mg/m^2/day, 2 patients with acute

TABLE 1. *AMSA therapy in patients with leukemia*

Dosage level (mg/m^2/day)	No. of patients	No. of courses	Toxicity	Response
1.3	1	1	0	0
5.0	1	1	0	0
30	2	6	0	1
40	3	6	0	1
100	4	7	0	2
125	6	10	4	5
150	7	13	4	4
Total	24	44	8	13

myelogenous leukemia (AML) of the 5 patients treated at these levels had marked reductions in leukocyte counts after three to four courses of AMSA, 53,000 to 2,700 and 179,000 to 5,000, respectively, but both patients had persistent M-3 marrows. Two of 4 patients treated with 100 mg/m^2/day (1 patient with ALL and 1 patient with AML) had reductions in leukocyte counts and disappearance of circulating blast cells; these effects were achieved following only one course of chemotherapy, but, similarly, marrow examinations disclosed M-3 status. Five of 6 patients who received 125 mg/m^2/day for 5 days responded to treatment. Within 5 days, 2 of the responders who had T-cell ALL had decreases in leukocyte counts from 194,000 and 136,000 to 900 and 1,000, respectively. In addition, 1 of these patients had more than 50% reduction in size of spleen and complete disappearance of a left pleural effusion. Two other responders had AML with clearing of circulating blasts, and 1 patient attained an M-2 marrow. The 5th responder at this dosage level was a patient with non-Hodgkin's lymphoma with marrow involvement who had complete regression of cervical lymphadenopathy, an anterior chest wall mass, and disappearance of the tumor cells in the marrow. Finally, of the 7 patients who received the highest dosage level of 150 mg/m^2/day, 4 patients (2 with T-cell ALL) had marked reduction in size of tumoral masses and/or reduction in levels of circulating blasts as evidence of antileukemic activity. One patient with ALL achieved an M-1 marrow. The responses at this dosage level occurred following only one course of AMSA administration.

Patients with Solid Tumors

Thirty courses of AMSA at six different dosage levels were given to the 17 patients with solid tumors (Table 2). Toxicity did not occur until the dosage level of 20 mg/m^2/day for 5 days when 1 of 2 patients developed moderate leukopenia with 1,300 white blood count/mm^3. The next 2 patients treated with 25 mg/m^2/day for 5 days experienced no toxicity; however, all 7 patients treated with 50 mg/m^2/day for 5 days developed toxic effects. Five patients had reversible myelosuppression (4 patients, leukopenia, 1,600 to 1,900 cells/mm^3; 4 patients, anemia, 7.3 to 8.2 g/dl). Two patients experienced vomiting, and 1 patient each had stomatitis and phlebitis. There were no oncolytic effects in this group of patients.

TABLE 2. *AMSA therapy in patients with solid tumors*

Dosage level (mg/m^2/day)	No. of patients	No. of courses	Toxicity
5.0	2	3	0
10	2	4	0
15	2	3	0
20	2	4	1
25	2	4	0
50	7	12	7
Total	17	30	8

DISCUSSION

This study was designed to define the minimum toxic dosages and the maximum tolerated dosages of AMSA in children with refractory forms of cancer. Interestingly, we observed that the minimum toxic dosage differed in pediatric patients with leukemia and solid tumors. In the former group, the first dosage at which toxic effects were observed in the daily-for-5-days schedule was 125 mg/m^2/day; in patients with solid tumors, toxicity was initially seen when less than one-fifth of that dosage was given (20 mg/m^2/day for 5 days). Likewise, the maximum dosage used here in the solid tumor group was 50 mg/m^2/day when all patients developed toxicity. In contrast, in patients with leukemia, higher dosage levels could be given. In these patients, the maximum tolerated dosage was threefold higher (150 mg/m^2/day for 5 days) when dose-limiting stomatitis and vomiting developed. The reason for different tolerance to chemotherapy in patients with leukemia and solid tumors is unknown, but has been previously noted in other phase I studies conducted with pediatric subjects at our institution (4). Although it is possible that patients with solid tumors may tolerate higher dosages than 50 mg/m^2/day for 5 days, it is unlikely that these will be as high as the dosages tolerated by patients with leukemia.

The testing of new oncolytic agents is necessary in pediatric patients because drug toxicity may differ not only between patients with acute leukemia and solid tumors but also between adults and children. In fact, there are few antineoplastic drugs that undergo phase I evaluation in pediatric patients. In addition, children have different tumor types with different sensitivities to chemotherapy than do adults. Among tumors that can be studied in children and young adults are neuroblastoma, rhabdomyosarcoma, Ewing's sarcoma, osteosarcoma, the lymphomas, and acute leukemias. Although the dose-limiting forms of toxicities seen in adults and children may be similar, the maximum tolerated dosages are not always equivalent.

As with most phase I clinical trials, the starting dosage in this study was one-third of the toxic dosage low in large animals. In the daily-for-5-days schedule under investigation, the dosage corresponded to 1.3 mg/m^2/day. Initially, it was planned to escalate the dosage levels slowly from 1.3 to 20 mg/m^2/day; however, no biological activity could be detected until dosages were increased 20-fold for patients with solid tumors and 100-fold for patients with leukemia. As the study proceeded, escalations could be performed more rapidly because information from other ongoing phase I studies became available from investigators at the National Cancer Institute (6), Baltimore Cancer Research Center (5), and M.D. Anderson Hospital (3).

Although not the primary objective of a phase I trial, it was encouraging to note the effectiveness of this new agent. The study clearly demonstrated evidence of antileukemic effects following the administration of AMSA at dosage levels equal to or higher than 30 mg/m^2/day for 5 days. This finding is interesting, considering the late stages of disease in the subjects studied, all of whom had disease refractory to agents of established effectiveness. To attain a complete response (M-1 marrow)

other patients reported from Manchester, England (Bramwell, *personal communication*). One of these patients was treated with uridine eyedrops and received further PALA infusions without recurrence of conjunctivitis. The peak plasma concentration after a dose of 2.5 g/m² was of the order of 7×10^{-4} M dropping to 2×10^{-6} M at 24 hr. The patient previously described with a low creatinine clearance had a peak of 4.4×10^{-5} M at 24 hr. This patient's total body clearance after a 50% dose was 28 ml/min. The peak concentration after a 3-hr infusion was 6.1×10^{-4} with a 24-hr concentration of 2.2×10^{-6} M.

Pharmacokinetics

The data fitted a three-compartment model with half-life times in the order of 1 hr, 2.5 hr, and 9 hr. Urinary excretion paralleled plasma concentration. In 1 patient, saliva and sweat were collected and concentrations were below 5×10^{-7} M. Samples of tears were collected in another patient because of the reported conjunctivitis, and PALA was observed to be excreted with a tear/plasma concentration ratio of 0.3.

Mouse Study

The peak plasma concentration obtained in mice was 2.5×10^{-4} M (corrected for a dose of 0.05 g/kg in accordance with the patient data). The total body clearance was 0.3 ml/min, which was calculated to be a relative clearance of 16 ml/min/kg. This compares with the calculated relative clearance in patients with normal renal function of 1.3 ml/min/kg (the value in the single patient with impaired renal function was 0.56 ml/min/kg). The indication from this data is that the clearance of PALA is considerably faster in mice than in humans, although the difference in route of administration of the drug, i.v. versus i.p., must be taken into account.

Cell Culture Study

Growth inhibition by 50% was achieved in each cell line at different PALA concentrations. For the melanoma lines, the concentrations were 2×10^{-5} M for murine B16 melanoma compared to 4×10^{-5} M for IPC-48 human-derived melanoma. These figures contrast with 3×10^{-4} M for murine L1210 leukemia and 2×10^{-4} M for human CEM leukemia. PALA therefore was much more effective in both melanoma lines than in the leukemia lines. This was not due to differences in doubling times between the lines, which varied with respect to species rather than histologic origin as follows:

human melanoma, 24 ± 4 hr; leukemia, 29 ± 5 hr
mouse melanoma, 16 ± 3 hr; leukemia, 13 ± 2 hr

The effect of action of PALA proved to be both on RNA and DNA. ¹⁴C-Guanine incorporation into nucleic acids of L1210 cells was studied during 24-hr exposure to PALA and showed that the block of DNA synthesis preceded that of RNA synthesis. During the 24-hr period at four sampling times, DNA synthesis was always inhibited to a greater extent than RNA synthesis by PALA. It was of interest, therefore, that in reversing studies, deoxycytidine, in addition to uridine or cytidine, also blocked PALA toxicity. Uridine and cytidine at concentrations of 5×10^{-5} M completely reversed PALA toxicity up to 48 hr. Deoxycytidine provided protection for 24 hr at doses as high as 10^{-4} M. Thymidine, on the other hand, enhanced PALA toxicity at concentrations that, when used alone in the medium, did not cause inhibition of cell growth. Evidence of true synergy was therefore obtained, though the combination has yet to be tested on other cell lines.

DISCUSSION

The differential sensitivities of PALA on a variety of tumours poses an intellectual and perhaps practical puzzle. PALA is attractive as an antimetabolite because it acts early in the *de novo* pyrimidine synthesis pathway; it has interesting activity in solid tumours rather than in the usual screening L1210 leukemia; toxicity is not found in the bone marrow; and the possibility for a selective effect due to variations of biochemical activity from tissue to tissue exist. It is known that the enzyme that PALA inhibits, ATCase, is significantly lower in PALA-sensitive tumours compared to PALA-resistant tumours. Within the sensitive group, however, the degree of ATCase activity and the degree of sensitivity to PALA are not related in a linear fashion (2). Further, the degree of inhibition of nucleotides is slightly greater for some tumours than for normal tissue, such as spleen, or leukocytes. Of even more potential importance is the differential rate of recovery from PALA blockade which is, in most systems, to the advantage of normal host tissues. Cytosine nucleotides recover much faster in marrow tissue after exposure to PALA than do the same nucleotides measured in colonic tumours. Cytosine arabinoside, therefore, introduced at a critical time after PALA exposure, might cause selective damage to tumour in which there are less competing cytosine nucleotides. It has been shown above that thymidine given with PALA causes a synergistic antagonism in tumour cells. What has not yet been shown is if this is true also for normal tissue. Combination of PALA with other antimetabolites is also attractive. PALA has been shown to increase the incorporation of 5-fluorouracil into RNA in some tumour systems (5). PALA may also assist the effect of 5-fluorouracil by increasing intracellular phosphoribosyl pyrophosphate (PRPP) pools. Methotrexate has a similar effect on PRPP, which may be one explanation for the occasional synergism of methotrexate and 5-fluorouracil in certain cell lines.

Clearly, PALA as a single agent has yet to prove its clinical use. The contrast of action in man and mice has been shown in both our cell culture studies and in the pharmacokinetic study above. The mechanism of relative resistance of human tumours compared to murine tumours may lie purely in the pharmacokinetics of the drug, though this would seem unlikely to be the whole interpretation. Jayaram has shown that the degree of sensitivity does not seem to be related to the kinetics of inhibition of ATCase or its ability to recover after inhibition, nor does it depend on detoxification of PALA or the kinetics of possible rescue by endogenous uridine (1). It may be, however, that the kinetics of uridine uptake may differ from cell to cell and the availability of uridine may differ between species. A recent study has shown that the only responding patient out of 5 studied was the single patient whose plasma uridine level dropped most significantly during PALA exposure (3). It is possible that liver cells continuously produce uridine and are thus able in most patients to bypass the block of PALA by supplementing uridine levels. On the other hand, certain tumours may be able to utilize uridine better than normal tissues. The opportunity for high-dose PALA administration with selective rescue by uridine could be exploited. The pharmacokinetic studies shown here are in accord with others in the literature and, taken in combination with cell culture data, show that PALA is very slowly transported into cells (4). The drug could be given by infusion in high but tolerable doses and the potential for local rescue with uridine, either applied locally to the skin or in an oral preparation to protect the gut, seems worthy of further study.

CONCLUSION

PALA is more effective in mouse tumours than in clinical practice. It remains, however, a potential drug for biochemical manipulation of nucleotide metabolism, which could lead to rendering tumour cells vulnerable to a second antimetabolite.

REFERENCES

1. Jayaram, H. N., Cooney, D. A., Vistica, D. T., Kariya, S., and Johnson, R. K. (1979): Mechanisms of sensitivity or resistance of murine tumours to N-(phosphonacetyl)-L-asparate (PALA). *Cancer Treat. Rep.*, 63:1,291–1,302.
2. Johnson, R. K., Swyryd, E. A., and Stark, G. R. (1978): Effects of N-(phosphonacetyl)-L-aspartate on murine tumours and normal tissues *in vivo* and *in vitro*. *Cancer Res.*, 38:371–378.
3. Karle, J. M., Anderson, L. W., Ehrlichman, C., and Cysyk, R. L. (1980): Serum uridine levels in patients receiving PALA. *Cancer Res.*, 40:2,938–2,940.
4. Loo, T. L., Friedman, J., Moore, E. C., Valdivieso, M., Marti, J. R., and Stewart, D. (1980): Pharmacological disposition of PALA in humans. *Cancer Res.*, 40:86–90.
5. Nayak, R., Martin, D., Stolfi, R., Furth, J., and Spiegelman, S. (1978): Pyrimidine nucleosides enhance the anticancer activity of 5-FU and augment its incorporation into nuclear RNA. *Proc. Am. Assoc. Cancer Res.*, 19:63.

New Approaches in Cancer Therapy,
edited by H. Cortés Funes and M. Rozencweig.
Raven Press, New York © 1982.

Rationale for New Clinical Studies with Doxorubicin

Franco M. Muggia, James L. Speyer, and Joseph Bottino

Division of Oncology, Department of Medicine, New York University Medical Center, New York, New York 10016

Efforts are being made to develop new anthracycline antibiotics and synthetic deoxyribonucleic acid (DNA)-intercalating compounds (23) which may share in the therapeutic activity of doxorubicin without some of its toxicities. While these leads are being pursued in drug development, the therapeutic index of doxorubicin itself may perhaps be improved through conceptual and technical advances.

The idea that free radical damage accounts for doxorubicin cardiotoxicity and that it may be dose related (20) has led to testing of protective measures through (a) use of free radical scavengers, and (b) dose-schedule alterations that retain therapeutic efficacy while possibly avoiding toxic free radical reactions. New techniques of drug delivery (5) and noninvasive assessment of left ventricular function (4) permit testing of these new leads. Such studies promise not only to enhance the safety of current doxorubicin use but also to expand the prospects of using it in situations that are presently deemed unsafe. We review in this chapter the rationale and direction of clinical studies that we and others have begun with doxorubicin.

DOSE-SCHEDULE ALTERATIONS

A large retrospective review (26) has confirmed previous observations that more frequent administration of doxorubicin in lower individual doses was associated with a lesser risk of cardiotoxicity and a greater probability of exceeding the "conventional" cumulative dose levels of 550 mg/m^2 without resulting in cardiomyopathy. This suggests that peak levels of the drug could bear a relationship to cardiotoxicity; antitumor efficacy, on the other hand, is presumably related to administration of dosages that avoid high peak levels but expose the tumor to equivalent amounts of drug (areas under the curve of concentration × time). Accordingly, trials were begun at the M. D. Anderson Hospital that compared an every 3-week versus a weekly administration. Weekly schedules, however, possess the intrinsic practical disadvantages of inconvenience, enhanced chance of extravasation, and increased difficulties in venous access.

Various techniques for drug delivery via central venous catheters have recently been introduced (Table 1). These methods have permitted the testing of continuous infusion schedules of doxorubicin (Table 2). It is important to stress that, without

TABLE 1. *Central venous catheterization methods*

Access vein	Insertion technique	Acute technical complications	Comments
Subclavian (27)[a]	Blind percutaneous	Multiple—potentially fatal	Suitable for emergencies and long-term infusions
Internal jugular (9)	Blind percutaneous	Multiple—potentially fatal	Suitable for emergencies, inconvenient for long-term infusions
Distal cephalic/basilic (6)	Percutaneous	None serious	Suitable for long-term and ambulatory infusions
Proximal cephalic (7)	Cut-down and subcutaneous tunneling	None serious	Suitable for long-term and ambulatory infusions
Femoral (5)	Blind percutaneous	Few—potentially serious	Short-term infusions only

[a]Numbers in parentheses are references.

TABLE 2. *Doxorubicin continuous infusion regimens*

References	Regimen (infusion)	Dose	Comments
Montinari et al. (19)	30-min	75 mg/m²	"Less clinical cardiotoxicity observed"
Stewart et al. (25)	24–96 hr	Not stated	Sarcomas: given with cytoxan, vincristine, and DTIC[a]
Legha et al. (18)	24–96 hr	60–90 mg/m²	Breast cancer, CMF failures
Pouillart and Garcia Giral *(personal communication)*	24 hr	40–50 mg/m²	Breast cancer alone and in combination
Gercovich et al. (15)	10 hr	60–75 mg/m²	Twenty patients reported
Garnick et al. (14)	indefinite, continuous daily	1–9 mg/m²	Infusaid pump refilled weekly
Our studies	24 hr, 6 hr	60–90 mg/m² 60–90 mg/m²	

[a]DTIC = diethyl triazeno imidazole carboxamide.

these new practical means for access into high-flow venous systems, such schedules cannot be tested with doxorubicin because of the risk of peripheral extravasations and severe necrosis. In fact, previous explorations of doxorubicin infusions were limited to ½-hr infusions (19).

The efficacy of continuous infusions of doxorubicin appears to be retained, according to preliminary reports of its activity when used alone in breast cancer patients who have failed cytoxan methotrexate 5-fluorouracil (CMF) (18) and when used in combination in soft tissue sarcomas at the M. D. Anderson Hospital (25). Preliminary reports of studies concerning cardiotoxicity, on the other hand, have revealed a significant decrease in progression of endomyocardial changes with doses as recorded by the Stanford biopsy score (12).

We have carried out feasibility studies of continuous infusion of doxorubicin primarily by the femoral route. Initially, a 24-hr infusion was used in 39 patients (24). Results of this phase I investigation revealed predominantly dose-limiting hematologic toxicity in 11 of 34 patients at 60 mg/m^2 over 24 hr. Twenty-seven patients could be escalated to 75 mg/m^2 and 9 patients to 90 mg/m^2 before encountering myelosuppression. Other toxicities included mild nausea, rare vomiting, and universal alopecia.

The number of patients at risk due to high cumulative dose received was too small to indicate if cardiotoxicity was lessened; efficacy data cannot be adequately interpreted. Responses were seen in 3 of 6 patients with endometrial cancer; only 1 patient of 10 with lung cancer had an objective response. The study conclusively demonstrated, however, that the 24-hr infusion via the femoral route was practical and had few complications: 2 patients with pelvic disease did develop femoral thromboses. We have since begun a similar phase II/III study of 6-hr infusion because of the practical advantages of this relatively shorter interval.

It is too early to comment on results of 6-hr infusions, but we shall present some of the directions that these preliminary clinical studies will take.

FREE RADICAL SCAVENGERS AND OTHER PROTECTIVE MEASURES

Formation of semiquinone free radicals of doxorubicin and eventual generation of superoxide species under aerobic conditions have been demonstrated in a number of experimental systems (3,21). Doroshow et al. have postulated mediation of cardiotoxicity via formation of superoxide free radicals and inadequate enzymatic protection of the myocardium against these species (11). In mice, α-tocopherol was able to protect against cardiotoxic death under some, but not all, experimental conditions. Similar results have been obtained with N-acetylcysteine, another radical scavenger (10). Also, coenzyme Q-10 has been postulated to be protective (13), although experimental verification of protection against doxorubicin-induced cardiotoxicity is wanting.

In the rabbit, Bristow et al. (7) demonstrated that doxorubicin caused an acute release of histamine and catecholamines. Myocardial lesions could be prevented by histaminergic and adrenergic blockade. These studies, summarized in abstract form only (7), imply additional possibilities for protecting against doxorubicin cardiotoxicity, which might also be related to the favorable effect of dose-schedule alterations. Verification of these observations for humans and for tumor-bearing animals, however, is required before therapeutic trials can be considered.

A final observation about protection from cardiotoxicity concerns the known risk factor of concomitant radiation therapy. Hypotheses about protection from free radical damage extend to radiation-induced damage and its pathogenesis. Clinical circumstances in which both radiation therapy to the heart and doxorubicin are given must be avoided if possible. Breast cancer adjuvant programs are increasingly incorporating doxorubicin; therefore, the avoidance of extensive chest irradiation, which is occasionally still carried out, appears important.

NEW DIRECTIONS OF CLINICAL STUDIES

The capability of altering the cardiotoxicity of doxorubicin introduces new prospects for uses of the drug. Most studies have generally avoided use of doxorubicin as an adjuvant in breast cancer; when it has been used (8), the doses may have been suboptimal. Although avoidance of the risks of cardiotoxicity in an adjuvant situation seems sensible, it is known that, in advanced breast cancer, doxorubicin-containing combination chemotherapy is superior to combinations without this agent (28). Modification of cardiotoxicity would allow regimens such as fluorouracil-adriamycin-(doxorubicin)-cyclophosphamide (FAC) to be used in high-risk groups after mastectomy. Accordingly, we have begun a protocol of infusion of FAC to define the cardiotoxic potential of this combination with doxorubicin as a 6-hr infusion (Table 3). Similarly, more aggressive adjuvant therapy may be considered in soft tissue sarcomas. Effectiveness of adjuvant therapy with doxorubicin relative to historical controls has been reported in trials at the National Cancer Institute and The Sidney Farber Center Institute (2,22). However, the technique of gated pool scans, including determination of ejection fraction (EF) after exercise, has revealed a greater than 50% incidence of cardiac function abnormalities (16). These considerations make it imperative that the therapeutic index of anthracyclines be improved by modification of cardiomyopathy.

In advanced malignancies, doxorubicin treatment is often discontinued before achievement of complete response or while efficacy is retained. This is done at a cut-off point of a cumulative dose of 550 mg/m^2 or lower because of the reported increase in the incidence of cardiotoxicity above this level (26). The continuation of doxorubicin treatment beyond 550 mg/m^2 may improve therapeutic results in lymphomas, leukemias, breast cancer, sarcomas, small cell carcinomas of the lung, and others. Finally, many patients are currently excluded from receiving anthracyclines because of age or heart disease. Improved outlook for prostate and endometrial cancer may result if doxorubicin could be applied to more patients or in full therapeutic doses. In both these conditions, found predominantly in the elderly, doxorubicin has demonstrated activity but is often withheld for fear of complications. In our phase II infusion studies in these conditions, we are including patients with prior heart disease—feasible as long as careful observations by cardiac monitoring can be carried out. Radionucleide-'gated' angiography allows the measurement of left ventricular EF and serial follow-ups (1,4). The response of this EF to exercise appears to be a most sensitive indicator of cardiomyopathy.

TABLE 3. *NYU Chemotherapy protocol for advanced breast cancer (Jan. 1981)*

Adriamycin, 50 mg/m^2, 6-hr infusion, d.l
Cyclophosphamide, 500 mg/m^2, d.l
5-Fluorouracil, 500 mg/m^2, d.l, 8, repeat every 21 days
No prior chemo Rx
Baseline gated pool scan
Repeat gated pool scan at 200 mg/m^2, 500 mg/m^2, and every other cycle thereafter

In conclusion, conceptual and technical advances are permitting studies designed to improve the therapeutic index of doxorubicin. These studies hold as much promise as the development of new analogs, and should be carried out in academic centers where clinical investigations with the participation of persons with highly developed specialties are possible.

ACKNOWLEDGMENTS

Supported in part by The Lila Motley Fund of New York University and by a grant from The Chemotherapy Foundation.

REFERENCES

1. Alexander, J., Dainiak, N., Berger, H., Goldman, L., Johnston, D., Reduto, L., Duffy, T., Schwartz, P., Gottschalk, A., and Zaret, B. (1979): Serial assessment of cardiac performance with quantitative radionucleide angiography. *N. Engl. J. Med.*, 300:278–283.
2. Antman, K., Blum, R., Corson, J., Wilson, R., Greenberger, J., Ash, A., and Frei, E. (1980): Effective adjuvant chemotherapy for localized soft tissue sarcoma. *Proc. Am. Assoc. Cancer Res.*, 21:565.
3. Bachur, N. (1979): Anthracycline antibiotic pharmacology and metabolism. *Cancer Treat. Rep.*, 63:817–820.
4. Borer, J., Bacharach, S., Green, M., Kent, K., Epstein, S., and Johnston, G. (1977): Real-time radionucleide cineangiography in the noninvasive evaluation of global and regional left ventricular function at rest and during exercise in patients with coronary artery disease. *N. Engl. J. Med.*, 296:839–844.
5. Bottino, J., Levin, M., Hymes, K., Povillart, P., Muggia, F., and Nidus, B. (1980): Femoral venous cannulation for continuous adriamycin and vindesine infusions. *Cancer Immunol. Immunother. (Suppl.)*, 10:A22.
6. Bottino, J., McCredie, K. B., Groschel, D. H. M., and Lawson, K. (1979): Long-term intravenous therapy with peripherally inserted silicone elastomer central venous catheters in patients with malignant diseases. *Cancer*, 43:1,937–1,943.
7. Bristow, M., Billingham, M., and Daniels, J. (1979): Histamine and catecholamines mediate adriamycin cardiotoxicity. *Proc. Am. Assoc. Cancer Res.*, 20:477.
8. Buzdar, A., Blumenschein, G., Hortobagyi, G., and Yap, H. (1980): Five-year follow-up of FAC-BCG therapy of stage II and III breast cancer. *Cancer Immunol. Immunother. (Suppl.)*, 10:29.
9. Daily, P. O., Randall, B. G., and Shumway, D. E. (1970): Percutaneous internal jugular vein cannulation. *Arch. Surg.*, 101:534–536.
10. Doroshow, J., Locker, C., and Myers, C. (1979): The prevention of doxorubicin cardiac toxicity by N-acetylcysteine. *Proc. Am. Assoc. Cancer Res.*, 20:1,035.
11. Doroshow, J., Locker, C., and Myers, C. (1980): Enzymatic defenses of the mouse heart against reactive oxygen metabolites—Alterations produced by doxorubicin. *J. Clin. Invest.*, 65:128–135.
12. Ewer, M., Ali, M., Mackay, B., Wallace, S., Valdevieso, M., Legha, S., Tenczynski, I., and Benjamin, R. (1981): A comparison of cardiac biopsy grades and ejection fraction estimations in patients receiving adriamycin. *Proc. Am. Soc. Clin. Oncol.*, 22:C135.
13. Folkers, K., Choe, J., and Combs, A. (1978): Rescue by coenzyme Q from electrocardiographic abnormalities caused by the toxicity from adriamycin in the rat. *Proc. Natl. Acad. Sci.*, 75:5,178–5,180.
14. Garnick, M., Weiss, G., Steele, G., Israel, M., Barry, W., Billingham, M. Sack, M., Schade, G., Canellos, G., and Frei, E. (1981): Phase 1 trial of long-term continuous adriamycin administration. *Proc. Am. Soc. Clin. Oncol.*, 22:C106.
15. Gercovich, F., Praga, C., Beretta, G., Morgenfeld, M., Muchnik, J., Pesce, R., Ho, D., and Benjamin, R. (1979): Ten-hour continuous infusion of adriamycin. *Proc. Am. Soc. Clin. Oncol.*, 20:C337.
16. Gottdeiner, J., Mathison, D., Borer, J., Bono, R., Myers, C., Barn, L., Schwartz, P., Bacharach, S., Green, M., and Rosenberg, S. Doxorubicin cardiac toxicity: Assessment left ventricular dysfunction by radionucleide cineangiography. *Ann. Int. Med.*, 94:430–435.

17. Hickman, R. O., Buckman, C. D., Clift, R. A., Sanders, J. E., and Stewart, P. (1979): A modified right atrial catheter for access to the venous systems in marrow transplant recipients. *Surg. Gynecol. Obstet.*, 148:871–875.
18. Legha, S., Benjamin, R., Yap, H., and Freireich, E. (1979): Augmentation of adriamycin's therapeutic index by prolonged continuous i.v. infusion for advanced breast cancer. *Proc. Am. Assoc. Cancer Res.*, 20:A1,059.
19. Montinari, F., Tedeschi, L., Clerici, M., Fraschini, P., Beretta, G., and Luporini, G. (1980): Cardiotossicita da doxorubicina (ADR) infusionale: Oncologia Medica, Ospedale San Carlo Borromeo Via Pio Secondo, 3-20153 Milano. *Tumori*, 66:178.
20. Myers, C. E., McGuire, W. P., Liss, R. H., Ifrim, I., Grotzinger, K., and Young, R. C. (1977): Adriamycin: The role of lipid peroxidation in cardiac toxicity and tumor response. *Science*, 197:165–167.
21. Pietronigro, D., McGuiness, J., Koren, M., Crippa, R., Seligman, M., and Demopoulos, H. (1979): Spontaneous generation of adriamycin semiquinone radicals at physiologic pH. *Physiol. Chem. Phys.*, 11:405–414.
22. Rosenberg, S. A., and Sindelar, W. (1980): Surgery and adjuvant radiation-chemo-immuno in soft tissue sarcomas: Results of treatment of the NCL. In: *Therapeutic Progress in Ovarian Cancer, Testicular Cancer, and the Sarcomas,* edited by A. J. Van Oosterom, F. M. Muggia, and F. Cleton, pp. 397–413. Leiden University Press, The Netherlands.
23. Rozencweig, M., De Sloover, C. D., Von Hoff, D. D., Tagnon, H. J., and Muggia, F. M. (1979): Introduction: Anthracycline derivatives in new drug development. *Cancer Treat. Rep.*, 63:807–808.
24. Speyer, J. L., Bottino, J., Nidus, B., Blum, R., Wernz, J., Levin, M., Hymes, K., and Muggia, F. (1981): Adriamycin 24-hour infusion: A phase 1 trial. *Proc. Am. Soc. Clin. Oncol.*, 22:C122.
25. Stewart, D., Benjamin, R., Baker, L., Yap, B., and Bodey, G. (1980): New drugs for the treatment of soft tissue sarcomas. In: *Therapeutic Progress in Ovarian Cancer, Testicular Cancer, and Soft Tissue Sarcomas*, edited by A. Van Oosterom, F. Muggia, and F. Cleton, pp. 453–481. Leiden University Press, The Netherlands.
26. Von Hoff, D., Layard, M., Basa, P., Davis, H., Von Hoff, A., Rozencweig, M., and Muggia, F. (1979): Risk factors for doxorubicin-induced congestive heart failure. *Ann. Int. Med.*, 91:710–717.
27. Wilmore, D. W., and Dudrick, S. J. (1969): Safe long-term venous catheterization. *Arch. Surg.*, 98:252–258.
28. Young, R., Lippman, M., DeVita, V., Bull, J., and Tormey, D. (1977): Perspectives in breast cancer: 1976. *Ann. Int. Med.*, 86:784–798.

New Approaches in Cancer Therapy,
edited by H. Cortés Funes and M. Rozencweig.
Raven Press, New York © 1982.

VM-26 Therapy in Children with Drug-Refractory Lymphocytic Leukemia

Gaston Rivera, Gary V. Dahl, Sharon B. Murphy, W. P. Bowman, R. J. Aur, Thomas L. Avery, and J. V. Simone

St. Jude Children's Research Hospital, Memphis, Tennessee 38101

Despite modern chemotherapy, about ½ of children treated for acute lymphoblastic leukemia (ALL) relapse, either during or after the treatment course (2). The reasons for this circumstance almost always can be traced to the failure of chemotherapy to eradicate or permanently suppress all leukemia cells. This is especially so for patients whose leukemia is biologically disposed to the rapid development of drug resistance. Different combinations and higher dosages of previously used antileukemic drugs induce new remissions, but these are generally brief, giving way to progressively more resistant disease. At St. Jude Children's Research Hospital, phase I and 2 trials of potentially valuable antileukemic agents are conducted in patients with drug-refractory lymphocytic leukemias. We report in this chapter a series of such investigations with the podophyllum compound VM-26 (see Table 1), a semisynthetic derivative of the May-apple plant *(Podophyllum peltatum)*. First used in clinical trials in the early 1970s (4,9), VM-26 has major cytotoxic activity in mitosis (17) as well as the premitotic interval (8) of the cell cycle. The oncolytic effects of this compound and its congener, VP-16-213, were assessed in a preliminary study in patients with advanced unresponsive leukemia who had experienced multiple bone marrow relapses.

PHASE I STUDIES

As single agents, the epipodophyllotoxins induced objective responses in 9 of 29 children evaluated; most important, they were effective after established drugs

TABLE 1. *Clinical trials of VM-26 in childhood leukemia*

Treatment[a]	No. of patients	Clinical status of leukemia	Responses	CR[b]
VM-26 (or VP-16)	29	Advanced	9 (0.31)	0
VM-26 + ara-C	33	Advanced	10 (0.30)	9 (0.27)
VM-26 + ara-C	26	Second remission	Median 7 months	
VM-26 + ara-C	14	Induction failures	9 (0.64)	9 (0.64)
VM-26 + P + VCR	53	Advanced	26 (0.49)	17 (0.32)

[a]P: prednisone; VCR: vincristine.
[b]CR: complete remission.

had lost any demonstrable oncolytic activity. In responding patients, rapid reductions in leukocyte counts of 80% or more, with clearing of circulating lymphoblasts and a decrease in the proportion of bone marrow lymphoblasts (>50%), as well as disappearance of large tumor masses or malignant effusions, were observed. These results, defined as "oncolytic responses," provided evidence of a rapid antileukemic effect. With this single-drug therapy, however, no complete marrow remissions were induced. In addition to providing a clear indication that this new class of agents was active in children with refractory lymphocytic leukemia, the initial trials demonstrated that the epipodophyllotoxins could be administered without producing prohibitive toxicity. Myelosuppression was the most pronounced side effect produced by either VM-26 or VP-16-213 but, in general, was no more severe than that induced by most other antileukemic drugs (10). Bleyer and co-workers (1) reported similar results in subsequent phase II studies.

EARLY RESULTS OF COMBINATION CHEMOTHERAPY

As with most drugs, the epipodophyllotoxins have increased antitumor effects when used in combination. In animal studies with L1210 murine leukemia performed at our institution, VM-26 and cytosine arabinoside (ara-C) acted synergistically in curing or extending the life-spans of leukemic mice (11). By analysis of variance, the basis of the enhanced effect appeared to be a potentiation of ara-C activity by VM-26; this information, together with the performance of the podophyllotoxin in phase I studies, formed a rationale for using combinations of the two agents in patients with ALL for whom all other therapeutic possibilities had been exhausted.

The regimen was given initially to 33 children with multiple hematologic relapses (12). Because there was inadequate information on the use of VM-26 in combination chemotherapy for human subjects, the treatment design incorporated five increasing dosages of VM-26 (50, 75, 110, 165, or 200 mg/m^2/dose) combined with a constant dosage of ara-C (300 mg/m^2/dose). Each dosage combination was given twice a week for 4 weeks (total of eight doses). The initial dosage of VM-26, 50 mg/m^2/dose, furnished a basis for comparison of results of the previous single-drug study. The podophyllum compound was administered in 30- to 45-min i.v. infusions at a concentration of 1 mg/ml in a solution of 5% glucose and normal saline (1/3 dilution) to prevent crystallization. Ara-C was diluted to a final concentration of 50 mg/ml and administered by rapid i.v. injection immediately after the VM-26 infusion. No other antileukemic drugs were used for remission induction; antimicrobial agents, transfusions or blood products, and general supportive care were provided as required.

Ten of the 33 patients attained remissions (9 complete and 1 partial). Of the 23 nonresponders, 9 could not complete the study owing to their debilitated physical condition. Drug-induced toxicity was noted over the full range of VM-26 dosage; again, myelosuppression was the most frequent and most severe side effect observed. It occurred at each level of dosage, but was most prolonged at 200 mg/m^2, with 3, rather than 2, weeks required for hematologic recovery.

An optimally effective dosage of VM-26 for combination with ara-C was not clearly established by this study; instead, remissions were induced over the entire range of podophyllotoxin dosage (total dosages of 325 to 1,320 mg/m^2 versus 400 to 1,600 mg/m^2 for patients who failed to respond). Because the independent contribution by VM-26 in combination therapy is likely to be dosage dependent, we suggest that the drug be used at maximally tolerated dosage. In view of the more protracted myelosuppression after treatment with 200 mg/m^2, that dosage appears to be equal to or greater than 165 mg/m^2 but less than 200 mg/m^2.

This trial demonstrated that combinations of VM-26 and ara-C will induce complete remissions in a relatively high proportion of children with drug-refractory leukemia. Significantly, since 7 of 10 responders had previously received ara-C in other drug combinations, its prior use did not appear to diminish the effectiveness of the combination. Explanations for the therapeutic efficacy of this combination are still being sought, but, from available evidence, our working hypothesis is that oncolytic contributions are made by each of the drugs with ara-C activity being potentiated by VM-26.

Clinical studies to evaluate potentially useful antileukemic drugs have undergone major changes over the past 15 years. For example, when vincristine and daunomycin were first studied, the median duration of complete remissions was only approximately 1 year and prior chemotherapy was limited to only a few effective agents (7,8). In some instances, moreover, children who received these drugs were previously untreated (6). The patients admitted to this trial, by contrast, had shown clinical resistance to all first-line chemotherapy, including prednisone, vincristine, daunomycin, and asparaginase. Therefore, the induction of complete responses in about ⅓ of these children was encouraging, especially when one considers that 10 patients did not complete a full course of therapy and may have become responders had they been treated under more favorable circumstances.

In earlier evaluations of VM-26 and VP-16-213, neither compound proved therapeutically superior to the other; their toxic effects were comparable and both appeared to potentiate responses to ara-C in mice. Hence, the selection of VM-26 for combined drug treatment of ALL was arbitrary and should not be construed to indicate any superiority of this agent over its congener.

VM-26 AND ARA-C AS CONSOLIDATION THERAPY

A particularly difficult group of patients to treat are children who, after an initial bone marrow relapse during therapy, attain second remission. Generally, these remissions are short lived and many therapeutic efforts to prolong their duration have been unsuccessful (3,5,15). A comparative study was therefore designed to determine if a brief intensive treatment with VM-26 plus ara-C, after the reinduction of remission, would extend the duration of second hematologic remission in childhood ALL (13). To test this hypothesis, at the date of second remission we randomized patients to receive or not to receive four doses of VM-26 (165 mg/m^2) and ara-C (300 mg/m^2) over 2 weeks. Both treatment groups were comparable with respect to (a) prognostic features at diagnosis, (b) development of a first marrow relapse during a similar initial treatment, and (c) length of first marrow remission. In addition, all patients received identical reinduction therapy (prednisone, vincristine, daunomycin) and continuation therapy (weekly i.v. injections of vincristine and cyclophosphamide for 30 months plus intrathecal chemotherapy every 6 weeks). Thirty patients were randomized not to receive VM-26 plus ara-C, and their median duration of second remission was 3 months (1 to 16 months). Only 7 of 30 had prolonged second remissions (>6 months) and none were taken off chemotherapy. By comparison, 26 children were randomized to receive VM-26 + ara-C consolidation treatment, and their median duration of second remission was 7 months (2 to 47+ months), a significantly longer interval ($p = 0.04$) by logrank analysis. In this group, 14 of 26 children had prolonged second remissions and 2 are now off therapy, for 20+ and 22+ months, respectively, after successfully completing 30 months of continuation treatment. Reversible myelosuppression but no other untoward effects was observed in 25 of 26 patients treated with VM-26 and ara-C. Analysis of selected patient variables in this study indicated a clear correlation of early VM-26 + ara-C therapy with length of second remission. We concluded, then, that VM-26 + ara-C significantly extended the duration of second remissions. Furthermore, in 2 of these patients, treatments were electively stopped an unusual event following a marrow relapse on therapy.

VM-26 AND ARA-C FOR INDUCTION FAILURES

Lastly, a study was conducted in patients with ALL who failed to respond to initial induction therapy (induction failures) (14). There were 14 newly diagnosed patients who did not attain remission following 6 to 12 weeks of treatment with prednisone, vincristine, daunomycin, and asparaginase with or without ara-C. Nine of these patients had high-risk features at diagnosis, 6 had leukocyte counts exceeding 100,000 cells/mm^3, 6 had early CNS leukemia, and 5 had E-rosette-positive lymphoblasts. However, despite the presenting clinical and laboratory findings, each of the 14 patients had not attained an initial remission and consequently had a dire prognosis. The treatment plan for this group consisted of 4 weeks of combination chemotherapy with VM-26 at a 165 mg/m^2/dose and ara-C at a 300 mg/m^2/dose twice weekly. Three children did not respond and died; 2 responded, but did not attain remission and died; 9 attained complete remission. Of these 9 patients, 5 had clinical high-risk features at diagnosis, 3 had T-cell leukemia, and 6 had received previous ara-C therapy. Three of the 9 responders are still in remission, 2 off therapy for 26+ months and surviving 5 years after diagnosis. In this study, the complete remission rate was 64%, providing firm evidence that the effectiveness of the drug combination could be extended to newly diagnosed unresponsive patients.

VM-26, PREDNISONE, AND VINCRISTINE COMBINATION

To further exploit its therapeutic potential, we combined VM-26 with prednisone and vincristine (16). Only patients in relapse who had repeatedly received prednisone and vincristine were studied; the objective was to determine if drug synergism could be elicited with agents other than ara-C. Fifty-three patients with equally refractory lymphocytic leukemia were studied; 26 children responded to therapy, with 17 attaining complete marrow remission. These results indicated that responses to VM-26 therapy did not depend on the drug's combination with ara-C and, indirectly, provided evidence to suggest that clinical resistance to a compound or combination of compounds may be overcome by adding an effective new drug, such as VM-26, that has pronounced oncolytic activity and a different mechanism of antitumor activity.

CONCLUSION

The information from these trials should aid in the design of future treatment strategies for leukemia patients at high risk of early relapse. Since VM-26 in combination chemotherapy effectively destroyed populations of leukemia cells not susceptible to the cytotoxic activity of conventional agents, its most important future role may be in alternate remission induction treatments or, perhaps, as an added component of primary treatments.

ACKNOWLEDGMENTS

We thank John Gilbert for editorial assistance.

REFERENCES

1. Bleyer, W. A., Krivit, W., Chard, R. L., and Hammond, D. (1979): Phase II study of VM-26 in acute leukemia, neuroblastoma, and other refractory childhood malignancies: A report from the Children's Cancer Study Group. *Cancer Treat. Rep.*, 63:977–981.
2. Bowman, W. P. (1981): Childhood acute lymphocytic leukemia: Progress and problems in treatment. *Can. Med. Assoc. J.*, 124:129–142.
3. Chessells, J. M., and Cornbleet, M. (1979): Combination chemotherapy for bone marrow relapse in childhood lymphoblastic leukemia (ALL). *Med. Pediatr. Oncol.*, 6:359–365.
4. Dombernosky, P., Nissen, N. I., and Larsen, V. (1972): Clinical investigation of a new podophyllum derivative, epipodophyllotoxin, 4'-demethyl-9-(4,6-0-2-thenylidene-β-D-glucopyranoside) (NSC-122819), in patients with malignant lymphomas and solid tumors. *Cancer Chemother. Rep.*, 56:71–82.
5. Ekert, H., Ellis, W. M., Waters, K. D., and Matthews, R. N. (1979): Poor outlook for childhood acute lymphoblastic leukaemia with relapse. *Med. J. Aust.*, 2:224–226.
6. Evans, A. E., Farber, S., Brunet, S., and Mariano, P. J. (1963): Vincristine in the treatment of acute leukemia in children. *Cancer*, 16:1,302–1,306.
7. Karon, M., Freireich, E. J., Frei, E., III, Taylor, R., Wolman, I. J., Djerassi, I., Lee, S. L., Sawitsky, A., Hananian, J., Selawry, O., James, D., George, P., Patterson, R. B., Burgert, O., Haurani, F. I., Oberfield, R. A., Macy, C. T., Hoogstraten, B., and Blom, J. (1966): The role of vincristine in the treatment of childhood acute leukemia. *Clin. Pharmacol. Ther.*, 7:332–339.
8. Krishan, A., Paika, K., and Frei, E., III (1975): Cytofluorometric studies on the action of podophyllotoxin and epipodophyllotoxins (VM-26, VP-16-213) on the cell cycle traverse of human lymphoblasts. *J. Cell Biol.*, 66:521–530.
9. Mathé, G., Schwarzenberg, L., Pouillart, P., Weiner, R., Oldham, R., Jasmin, C., Rosenfeld, C., Hayat, M., Scheineder, M., Annel, J. L., Ceoara, B., Steresco-Nusset, M., and de Vassal, F. (1974): Essai de traitement de divers hematosacromes par le 4'-déméthyl-épipodophyllotoxine-beta-D-thénylidène glucoside (VM-26 or EPT). *Nouv. Presse. Med.*, 3:447–451.
10. Rivera, G., Avery, T., and Pratt, C. (1975): 4'-demethylepipodophyllotoxin 9-(4,6-0-2-thenylidene-β-D-glucopyranoside (NSC-122819; VM-26) and 4'-demethylepipodophyllotoxin 9-(4,6-0-

ethylidene-β-D-glucopyranoside) (NSC-141540; VP-16-213) in childhood cancer: Preliminary observations. *Cancer Chemother. Rep.*, 59:743–749.

11. Rivera, G., Avery, T., and Roberts, D. (1975): Response of L1210 to combinations of cytosine arabinoside and VM-26 or VP-16-213. *Eur. J. Cancer*, 11:639–647.

12. Rivera, G., Aur, R. J., Dahl, G. V., Pratt, C. B., Wood, A., and Avery, T. (1980): Combined VM-26 and cytosine arabinoside in treatment of refractory childhood lymphocytic leukemia. *Cancer*, 46:1,284–1,288.

13. Rivera, G., Dahl, G. V., Bowman, W. P., Aur, R. J. A., Murphy, S. B., and Tsiatis, A. (1981): Prolonged second marrow remission in children with lymphocytic leukemia (ALL) treated with VM-26 and cytosine arabinoside (Ara-C). *Proc. AACR and ASCO (Abstract)*, 22:481.

14. Rivera, G., Dahl, G. V., Bowman, W. P., Avery, T. L., Wood, A., and Aur, R. J. (1980): VM-26 and cytosine arabinoside combination chemotherapy for initial induction failures in childhood lymphocytic leukemia. *Cancer*, 46:1,727–1,730.

15. Rivera, G., Murphy, S. B., Aur, R. J. A., Verzosa, M. S., Dahl, G. V., and Mauer, A. M. (1978): Recurrent childhood lymphocytic leukemia. Clinical and cytokinetic studies of cytosine arabinoside and methotrexate for maintenance of second hematologic remission. *Cancer*, 42:2,521–2,528.

16. Rivera, G., Murphy, S. B., Wood, A., Dahl, G. V., Bowman, W. P., and Aur, R. J. A. (1979): Combination chemotherapy with prednisone, vincristine, and the epipodophyllotoxin VM-26 for refractory childhood lymphocytic leukemia (ALL). *Blood (Abstract)*, 54:265a.

17. Stahelin, H., and Poschmann, G. (1978): Effects of the epipodophyllotoxin derivative VM-26 in mitosis and in interphase. *Oncology*, 35:217–219.

18. Tan, C., Tasaka, H., Yu, K. P., Murphy, M. L., and Karnofsky, D. (1967): Daunomycin, an antitumor antibiotic, in the treatment of neoplastic disease. *Cancer*, 20:333–353.

New Approaches in Cancer Therapy,
edited by H. Cortés Funes and M. Rozencweig.
Raven Press, New York © 1982.

VP-16-213 Plus 5-Azacytidine for Remission Induction of Refractory Acute Nonlymphocytic Leukemia

Gary V. Dahl, A. Thomas Look, and Gaston Rivera

St. Jude Children's Research Hospital, Memphis, Tennessee 38101

The proportion of patients with acute nonlymphocytic leukemia (ANLL) who respond to initial treatment has improved sufficiently so that now, complete remissions may be expected for 60 to 80% of newly diagnosed patients (8). Effective intensive combination chemotherapy with anthracyclines and cytosine arabinoside (ara-C) and better supportive care have been responsible for this level of success. Despite remission maintenance therapy with these and other agents, completed studies report a median remission duration of only 26 to 50 weeks (8). Depending on initial therapy, second remissions may be difficult to induce after relapse during chemotherapy; when this occurs, such patients inevitably become resistant to all known effective agents. The major problem in ANLL is, therefore, early relapse with drug-resistant disease. At St. Jude Hospital, we have developed a program to identify effective new drug combinations for primary therapy. The subjects of this program are the patients who relapse on first-line therapy.

The following study was designed to assess the therapeutic value of combining VP-16-213 (VP-16) with 5-azacytidine (5-AZ)—two drugs with proven activity in single-agent trials for refractory ANLL (20,24). VP-16 is a semisynthetic epipodophyllotoxin derivative that induces premitotic arrest of cell cycle progression *in vitro* and is most cytotoxic for cells in the S and G_2 phases (7,11). VP-16 has had demonstrable activity in previously treated patients with ANLL (19,24) and, in a recent trial, provided an 8% complete remission rate for 66 children with ANLL in relapse (4). 5-AZ is a pyrimidine nucleotide analog that can become incorporated into nucleic acids and interfere with ribonucleic acid (RNA) and deoxyribonucleic acid (DNA) synthesis (24). This drug has shown activity against ANLL in both adults and children (1,10,14); in a large cooperative trial (21), 5-AZ alone provided a 14% complete remission rate for 71 patients with ANLL in relapse. The study described in this chapter indicates that these two drugs, given in high dosages in an intensive schedule, may induce marrow hypoplasia and subsequent complete remissions in about ½ of patients with refractory ANLL.

MATERIALS AND METHODS

This study included 40 patients who relapsed during therapy or failed induction during the St. Jude AML-76 and AML-80 protocol studies for newly diagnosed patients with ANLL (1,6). The clinical characteristics and previous therapy for these patients is listed in Table 1. In accordance with the AML-76 protocol, patients received vincristine, daunomycin, 6-azauridine, and ara-C for remission induction. Continuation therapy consisted of monthly vincristine, cyclophosphamide, and adriamycin. During the intervening 3 weeks, daily 6-mercaptopurine and ara-C were given. Treatment was to continue for 30 months. In accordance with the AML-80 protocol, remission induction therapy was an intensive combination of daunomycin, given for 3 days, and continuous infusion of ara-C, given for 7 days (17). Thirty of the 40 patients were initially treated according to the AML-76 protocol, and 2 according to the AML-80 protocol. The remaining 8 patients had previously received various therapies that combined anthracyclines and ara-C. Before VP-16 and 5-AZ were given, 19 of 40 patients also had received reinduction therapy with methotrexate followed by asparaginase, as described by Capizzi and Dahl et al. (3,5). Two patients had failed to respond to 5-AZ as a single agent before they entered the current study.

Therapeutic Regimens

Patients with recurrent relapse disease or ANLL refractory to initial therapy were treated according to one of two regimens. The first 16 patients, entered between February 1978 and January 1979, received successive 5-day courses of VP-16 (100 mg/m^2 daily for 3 days) and 5-AZ (150 mg/m^2 daily for 2 days). Half of the patients received the three doses of VP-16 before the two doses of 5-AZ, and half received 5-AZ for 2 days before the doses of VP-16. Both groups received the same dosage of each drug per course, which was repeated after 9 to 16 days.

The next 24 patients, entered between February 1979 and April 1980, received a more intensive treatment with successive 5-day courses: VP-16 (200 mg/m^2) daily

TABLE 1. *Patient characteristics*

	Initial regimen	Intensive regimen
Total no. of patients	16 (10 males, 6 females)	24 (11 males, 13 females)
Median age in years (range)	13 (2–19)	12 (1–19)
ANLL type[a]		
Myelocytic (M1,M2)	12	13
Progranulocytic (M3)	1	1
Myelomonocytic (M4)	2	5
Monocytic (M5)	1	5
Treatment history		
Induction failure on primary therapy	4	5
First relapse	8	19
Two or more relapses	3	0
AML[b] as second cancer	1	0

[a]Classified according to the FAB Cooperative Group (2).
[b]AML = acute myelogenous leukemia.

for 3 days followed by 5-AZ (300 mg/m^2) daily for 2 days. To determine the effects of VP-16 on leukemic blast proliferation *in vivo*, we serially studied the bone marrow aspirates from 8 of these children—the subjects of an earlier report (13). For this more intensive treatment, the interval between courses was shortened to 1 to 2 days.

With either schedule, courses were repeated until marrow hypoplasia or progressive leukemia was documented. Once hypoplasia was achieved, chemotherapy was stopped and bone marrow aspirates were obtained each week to monitor marrow recovery. If leukemic blasts, rather than normal marrow cells, returned, 2 to 3 additional 5-day courses of chemotherapy were given.

Definition of Terms and Supportive Treatments

Marrow hypoplasia was defined as hypocellularity of the marrow aspirate with less than 5% total blast cells and no identifiable malignant blasts in two Wright stain smears. The criteria for complete remission were findings of a cellular marrow with active normal hematopoiesis, less than 5% blast cells and no definite leukemic blasts, and normal blood cell counts. Chemotherapy was administered in the outpatient clinic unless other treatment was required for infection or bleeding. Gentamicin and oxacillin (i.v.) were used empirically for fever with neutropenia. Packed red cell transfusions were given to maintain a hemoglobin of 8 to 10 g/100 ml. Platelet transfusions were not given prophylactically. However, platelet concentrates were used for bleeding associated with thrombopenia or for preventing central nervous system bleeding after mucosal or retinal hemorrhages developed. White blood cells obtained by continuous flow separation were transfused for documented gram-negative infections that did not respond to antibiotics alone. Total parenteral nutrition was given through a central venous catheter when weight loss exceeded 10% or when serum albumin was less than 3.5 g/100 ml in anorectic patients.

RESULTS

The effectiveness of the two therapy schedules was clearly different (Table 2). The initial regimen was ineffective; only 1 of 16 patients achieved marrow hypoplasia and complete remission. For patients in the initial treatment, the number of leukemic blasts in the blood frequently increased during the 1 to 2 weeks between courses, even though there was usually an initial decrease during and immediately following the 5-day treatment. Since progressive disease, rather than toxicity, was responsible for the therapy failure in 12 of the 16 patients given the initial regimen, two major modifications were made. The drug dosages were doubled and the interval between courses was decreased to 1 to 2 days. This intensification of therapy was intended to produce marrow hypoplasia quickly and to allow subsequent normal cell recovery. As shown in Table 2, these changes improved the effectiveness of this combination, since 19 of 24 patients had marrow hypoplasia and 11 of 24 patients achieved complete remission. The proportion of patients with hypoplasia

TABLE 2. *Efficacy of the two therapies*

	Initial regimen	Intensive regimen
Total no. of patients	16	24
No. with marrow hypoplasia and		
complete remission[a]	1	11
leukemic regrowth	0	7
death in hypoplasia	0	1
Subtotal	1	19
No. without response	12	3
No. who died during induction	3	2

[a]The proportion of patients who achieved complete remission and marrow hypoplasia was significantly greater for the intensive regimen [$p < 0.05$, Fisher's Test (12)].

and complete remission after the intensive treatment was significantly higher than that after the initial treatment ($p < 0.05$, Fisher's test) (12).

The patient on the initial regimen who achieved remission had acute myelocytic leukemia in first relapse and received two courses of therapy. Of the 11 patients on the intensive regimen who achieved remission, 8 had acute myelocytic leukemia, 1 had acute myelomonocytic and 2 had acute monocytic leukemia. To achieve remission, 5 patients required two courses, 4 patients required three courses, and 2 patients required four courses of chemotherapy. Three of these patients were induction failures of primary therapy and the remainder were in first hematologic relapse. Of the 12 patients who achieved complete remission, 5 received no further therapy and remained in remission for 12 to 29 weeks (median, 19 weeks), and 5 received monthly courses of VP-16 and 5-AZ and remained in remission for 1 + to 27 weeks (median, 11 weeks). The remaining 2 patients had bone marrow transplants shortly after achieving remission: 1 died of a cytomegalovirus infection 7 weeks following transplant and the other is still in remission following transplant in June 1979.

Toxicity

The major toxicity produced by the two drug regimens was prolonged pancytopenia that predisposed patients to infection and bleeding. With the initial schedule, neutropenia (<500/mm^3) and thrombopenia ($<30,000$/mm^3 or <2/oif) each developed in 15 of 16 patients. With a more intensive regimen, thrombopenia and neutropenia were present in all patients either when therapy was started or within the ensuing 13 days. The duration of pancytopenia was evaluated for patients who achieved complete remission with the intensive regimen. As shown in Table 3, the median interval between the start of therapy and the documentation of complete remission was 45 days. Neutropenia and thrombopenia persisted through most of this period (median durations were 36 and 38 days, respectively).

TABLE 3. *Hematologic recovery of 11 patients who achieved complete remission after intensive therapy*

	Median no. of days (range)
Interval from start of therapy to achievement of remission	45 (27–84)
Interval from end of therapy to achievement of remission	28 (14–49)
Duration of neutropenia (< 500 cells/mm^3)	36 (22–67)
Duration of thrombopenia ($< 30,000$ cells/mm^3)	38 (11–59)

Due to the prolonged period of pancytopenia, most patients had frequent episodes of serious bleeding and fever. On the initial regimen, 2 patients died of hemorrhage (1, generalized pulmonary, and the other, in the central nervous system). Another patient in the initial regimen died with documented gram-negative septicemia. With the intensive schedule, 2 patients died of central nervous system hemorrhage and 1 patient died of an upper gastrointestinal hemorrhage. Six who received the intensive treatment had documented bacteremia, 4 had localized cellulitis, 2 had pneumonia, 1 had Salmonella osteomyelitis, and 2 had Candida esophagitis that, in 1 patient, produced a tracheoesophageal fistula that required gastrostomy. Although infections were frequent, none of the patients on the intensive regimen died of this complication. Other toxic effects in all patients included alopecia and moderate to severe vomiting, often accompanied by diarrhea after 5-AZ infusions. Liver toxicity has been noted during single-agent trials with 5-AZ (24). Previous abnormalities of liver function in 3 patients were exacerbated by VP-16 and 5-AZ and contributed to the death of 2 of these patients. Four patients on the intensive regimen had reversible renal tubular dysfunction with hypochloremia, hyponatremia, hypomagnesemia, and hypocalcemia, as described in patients who received 5-AZ alone (15). This problem was reversible within 1 to 3 weeks.

Aggressive supportive care was necessary, particularly for the 24 patients on the intensive regimen. Twenty-two of these patients required hospitalization for broad spectrum antibiotic therapy after fever and neutropenia developed. The median duration of hospitalization was 21 days (range, 5 to 103 days). Five patients received white blood cell transfusions and all patients required platelet and red cell transfusions. Total parenteral nutrition was given to 6 patients. Despite this care, 4 patients died of hemorrhage associated with thrombopenia. Although infections were frequent, none were fatal.

DISCUSSION

Relapse with refractory disease is the hallmark of ANLL. The use of first-line agents for reinduction has been unsuccessful because these agents have been frequently used for maintenance of earlier remissions. Of prime importance is the development of new active combinations that can be used earlier during treatment to prevent subsequent recurrence.

VP-16 and 5-AZ, as combined in the intensive schedule, are effective for patients with ANLL who fail induction therapy or relapse during primary therapy that includes anthracyclines and ara-C. Our regimen was designed to produce marrow hypoplasia rapidly, with only 1 to 2 days between successive courses, and was superior to the less intensive regimen. The disappearance of leukemia cells and marrow hypoplasia are objective measures of the effect of chemotherapy on ANLL (9) and were evident in a significantly higher proportion of patients who received the intensive therapy (19 of 24 patients with versus 1 of 16 patients without intensive treatment, $p < 0.05$). In 11 of the 20 patients who responded, the reduction of leukemia cell numbers was sufficient to allow complete recovery of normal marrow function.

The two drugs were combined because they showed promise as single agents in pediatric patients (4,10,19). Based on the complete remission rate achieved with the intensive schedule of VP-16 and 5-AZ (11 of 24 patients), this combination appears to be one of the best alternatives available for ANLL that is refractory to first-line therapy. It is important to note that of the 5 patients who were resistant to primary induction therapy, 3 achieved complete remission with the intensive regimen.

The treatment for an individual patient at relapse depends on the specific drugs and drug regimens used for primary therapy. For patients who receive no maintenance chemotherapy during initial treatment, retreatment with the same drugs used for first remission induction appears most effective (23). The patients who fail induction therapy with first-line agents or who relapse despite intensive maintenance therapy should receive the intensive treatment with VP-16 and 5-AZ. The use of this drug combination during continuation therapy needs to be explored.

The success of reinduction therapy may heavily depend on the intensity of the drug regimen. This principle has been applied to most current schemes with anthracyclines and ara-C for inducing first remissions, and to the therapy design for patients who have shown primary drug resistance during therapy and are candidates for VP-16 and 5-AZ. Using the classification reported by Preisler (16), we determined that primary drug resistance was the principal reason that the initial regimen was ineffective; it accounted for 12 of 15 failures. When the drug dosages were increased in the intensive schedule, primary drug resistance could be overcome, since only 3 of 13 failures on the intensive schedule were due to primary resistance. Further support for the importance of combining these drugs in high dosages comes from the study of Van Echo and co-workers (22). Their treatment for ANLL in relapse consisted of courses of 5-AZ (150 mg/m^2) and VP-16 (75 mg/m^2) given daily for 5 days. The 14 patients treated according to this schedule did not achieve remission.

Due to the narrow therapeutic index of most active combinations in ANLL, prolonged pancytopenia and its associated infectious and bleeding complications represent a second hurdle in the way to remission induction. Prevention and control of these problems has allowed us to evaluate this intensive therapy with VP-16 and 5-AZ. The major complication expected of this therapy was prolonged pancytopenia.

The median time to achieve complete remission was longer than that reported for previously untreated patients who received anthracycline and ara-C. A median time of 33 days was required for patients to achieve remission when treated with adriamycin for 3 days and ara-C for 10 days (18). By comparison, the median period until complete remission in the VP-16 and 5-AZ intensive schedule was 45 days. Part of this delay was due to the increased time to deliver two to four courses of VP-16 and 5-AZ. However, there was also an increased time for marrow recovery after hypoplasia was documented and chemotherapy was stopped. With VP-16 and 5-AZ, the median delay of marrow recovery was 28 days after chemotherapy was stopped, compared to 19 days after a single course of adriamycin and ara-C (18). It is not surprising that the duration of marrow hypoplasia and pancytopenia was longer for our patients with refractory disease; many had received intensive chemotherapy before starting on this combination, so that some overlap of toxicity may have existed. Since all patients had received weeks to months of cytotoxic therapy prior to admission to our study, the number of marrow stem cells was probably decreased in this group of patients prior to VP-16 and 5-AZ therapy.

Unquestionably, in the past 10 years, there have been advances in the therapy for children with ANLL. While the proportion of patients responding to initial treatment was markedly improved, there has also been an increasing number of long remissions. As a result, 25 to 30% of those who achieve complete remission are projected to remain free of leukemia for more than 3 years. The major problem in ANLL is early relapse with drug-resistant disease. Therefore, it is important to develop more effective drug combinations that can be used earlier in therapy to prevent relapse. The development of a new drug combination for use as primary therapy is the basis of our study. The promising activity of the VP-16 and 5-AZ combination in refractory ANLL clearly indicates its potential for use in first-line chemotherapy protocols.

ACKNOWLEDGMENTS

We thank Jane Seifert for editorial assistance. Supported in part by Grants CA21765, CA20180, and CA15956 from the National Cancer Institute, the National Institutes of Health, and the Department of Health, Education, and Welfare, respectively, and by ALSAC.

REFERENCES

1. Baehner, R. L., Bernstein, I. D., Sather, H., Higgins, G., McCreadie, S., Chard, R. L., and Hammond, D. (1979): Improved remission induction rate with D-ZAPO but unimproved remission duration with addition of immunotherapy to chemotherapy in previously untreated children with ANLL. *Med. Pediatr. Oncol.*, 7:127–139.
2. Bennett, J. M., Catovsky, D., Daniel, M. T., Galton, D. A. G., Graenick, H. R., and Sultan, C. (1976): Proposals for the classification of the acute leukemias French-American-British (FAB) cooperative group. *Br. J. Haematol.*, 33:451–458.
3. Capizzi, R. L. (1975): Improvement in the therapeutic index of methotrexate by asparaginase. *Cancer Chemother. Rep.*, 6:37–41.

4. Chard, R. L., Jr., Krivit, W., Bleyer, W. A., and Hammond, D. (1979): Phase II study of VP-16-213 in childhood malignant disease: A Children's Cancer Study Group report. *Cancer Treat. Rep.*, 63:1,755–1,759.
5. Dahl, G., Amadori, S., Mason, C., Simone, J., and Aur, J. (1978): Methotrexate (MTX) followed in 24 hours by asparaginase (ASP) in childhood advanced acute nonlymphocytic leukemia (ANLL). *Proc. Am. Assoc. Cancer Res. (Abstract)*, 19:84.
6. Dahl, G. V., Murphy, S. B., Amadori, S., Simone, J. V., and Mauer, A. M. (1979): Sequential studies of marrow blast [^{3}H]thymidine-labeling indices (LI) during remission induction of acute nonlymphocytic leukemia (ANLL): An indicator for "high risk ANLL." *Blood*, 54 *(Suppl. 1)*: 185a.
7. Drewinko, B., and Barlogie, B. (1976): Survival and cycle-progression delay of human lymphoma cells *in vitro* exposed to VP-16-213. *Cancer Treat. Rep.*, 60:1,295–1,306.
8. Gale, R. P. (1979): Advances in the treatment of acute myelogenous leukemia. *N. Engl. J. Med.*, 300:1,189–1,199.
9. Galton, D. A. (1979): Can remission duration be prolonged in acute myeloid leukemia? *Recent Results Cancer Res.*, 69:55–62.
10. Karon, M., Sieger, L., Leimbrock, S., Finklestein, J. R., Nesbit, M. E., and Swaney, J. J. (1973): 5-Azacytidine: A new active agent for the treatment of acute leukemia. *Blood*, 42:359–365.
11. Krishan, A., Paika, K., and Frei, E., III (1975): Cytofluorometric studies on the action of podophyllotoxin and epipodophyllotoxins (VM-26,VP-16-213) on the cell cycle traverse of human lymphoblasts. *J. Cell Biol.*, 66:521–530.
12. Langley, R. (1970): *Practical Statistics*, pp. 292–317. Dover Publications, New York.
13. Look, T., Dahl, G., Murphy, S., and Mauer, A. (1980): Serial studies of the effects on blast cell kinetics of the epipodophyllotoxin VP-16-213 (VP-16) during the treatment of acute nonlymphocytic leukemia (ANLL). *Proc. Cell Kinet. Soc. (Abstract)*, 4:27.
14. McCredie, K. B., Bodey, G. P., Burgess, M. A., Rodriquez, V., Sullivan, M. P., and Freireich, F. (1972): The treatment of acute leukemia with 5-azacytidine. *Blood*, 40:975.
15. Peterson, B. A., Bloomfield, C. D., Vogelzang, N. J., and Collins, A. J. (1979): Renal tubular dysfunction during 5-azacytidine chemotherapy for acute leukemia. American Society of Hematology Meeting, Phoenix, Arizona. *Blood*, 54 *(Suppl. 1)*:202a.
16. Preisler, H. D. (1978): Failure of remission induction in acute myelocytic leukemia. *Med. Pediatr. Oncol.*, 4:275–276.
17. Preisler, H., Bjornsson, S., Henderson, E. S., Hryniuk, W., Higby, D., Freeman, A., and Naeher, C. (1979): Remission induction in acute nonlymphocytic leukemia: Comparison of a seven-day and ten-day infusion of cytosine arabinoside in combination with adriamycin. *Med. Pediatr. Oncol.*, 7:269–275.
18. Preisler, H., Rustum, Y., Henderson, E., Bjornsson, S., Creaven, P., Higby, D., Freeman, A., Gailani, S., and Naeher, C. (1979): Treatment of acute nonlymphocytic leukemia: Use of anthracycline-cytosine arabinoside induction therapy and comparison of two maintenance regimens. *Blood*, 53:455–464.
19. Rivera, G., Avery, T., and Pratt, C. (1975): 4'-Demethylepipodophyllotoxin 9-(4,6-0-2-thenylidene-β-D-glucopyranoside) (NSC-122819; VM-26) and 4'-demethylepipodophyllotoxin 9-(4,6-O-ethylidene-β-D-glucopyranoside) (NSC-141540; VP-16-213) in childhood cancer: Preliminary observations. *Cancer Chemother. Rep.*, 59:743–749.
20. Rozencweig, M., Von Hoff, D. D., Henney, J. E., and Muggia, F. M. (1977): VM-26 and VP-16-213: A comparative analysis. *Cancer*, 40:334–342.
21. Saiki, J. H., McCredie, K. B., Vietti, T. J., Hewlett, J. S., Morrison, F. S., Costanzi, J. J., Stuckey, W. J., Whitecar, J., and Hoogstraten, B. (1978): 5-Azacytidine in acute leukemia. *Cancer*, 42:2,111–2,114.
22. Van Echo, D. A., Lichtenfeld, K. M., and Wiernik, P. H. (1977): Vinblastine, 5-azacytidine, and VP-16-213 therapy for previously treated patients with acute nonlymphocytic leukemia. *Cancer Treat. Rep.*, 61:1,599–1,602.
23. Vaughan, W. P., Karp, J. E., and Burke, P. J. (1980): Long-term chemotherapy-free remissions after single-cycle timed sequential chemotherapy for acute myelocytic leukemia. *Cancer*, 45:859–865.
24. Von Hoff, D. D., Slavik, M., and Muggia, F. M. (1976): 5-Azacytidine: A new anticancer drug with effectiveness in acute myelogenous leukemia. *Ann. Intern. Med.*, 85:237–245.

New Approaches in Cancer Therapy,
edited by H. Cortés Funes and M. Rozencweig.
Raven Press, New York © 1982.

Treatment of Metastatic Nonseminomatous Testicular Cancer: A Preliminary Report of Induction Chemotherapy Followed by Maintenance Chemotherapy or Radiotherapy

*Roland W. Sonntag, **Hans Jörg Senn, and †Franco Cavalli

*Division of Oncology, University Clinics, Inselspital, 3010 Bern;
**Division of Oncology, Kantonsspital, 9006 St. Gallen; and
†Division of Oncology, Ospedale San Giovanni, 6500 Bellinzona, Switzerland*

Although significant advances in the treatment of nonseminomatous testicular carcinoma have been made during the past 18 years, the idea of possible curative management in the far-advanced metastatic stage of the disease is relatively new. As treatment improved through the availability of new and effective drugs, especially vinblastine (VBL) and bleomycin (BLM) (1), and the use of these agents in combination (2,6), remission rates of 60% to 80% were no longer uncommon. It also became obvious that only complete remissions (CR) were of benefit to the patient in terms of remission duration and survival (2,5,8), with a probability of cure approaching 50% (5,7).

In May 1976, the Swiss Group for Clinical Cancer Research (SAKK) initiated a study with two primary goals. The first was to achieve a high CR rate with an intensive polychemotherapy induction phase of treatment. A four-drug sequential program using two two-drug combinations was developed to permit higher dosage of the individual agents than would be possible if all four were given simultaneously. All four drugs had been of proven value in treating testicular carcinoma (1,4,7,9). The second goal was to determine the relative values of maintenance chemotherapy (MCT) versus radiation therapy (RT) for consolidation of these CR.

MATERIALS AND METHODS

All patients with histologically proven testicular carcinoma and radiologic or clinical evidence of inoperable metastases beyond the inguinal lymph nodes were eligible for the trial. Patients with pure seminomas were ineligible. Previous therapy could not have included any of the drugs used in the induction phase of treatment. Patients having previously received other drugs or RT were not excluded, provided that preexisting therapy-induced toxicity had fully subsided.

In addition to a complete physical examination, the following parameters were recorded at entry in the study: hemoglobin, platelet, leukocyte, and differential blood cell counts, urea nitrogen (BUN) or serum creatinine, alkaline phosphatase, serum glutamic oxaloacetic transaminase (SGOT), α-fetoprotein, serum or urine human chorionic gonadotropin, and chest roentgenogram. Liver scans or abdominal lymphangiograms were performed whenever indicated. All measurable tumor lesions were documented. The regular control of these parameters was defined in the protocol.

The induction program consisted of two sequential combination regimens (Fig. 1). The cis-dichlorodiammineplatinum (II) (cis platinum) dose was followed by forced diuresis (2,000 ml of glucose and saline infusion containing 40 g of mannitol and 40 mg of furosemide given over 6 to 8 hr). The adriamycin (ADM) and cis-platinum doses were each increased to 60 mg/m² after the first 21 evaluable patients showed only minimal hematologic toxicity and virtually no nephrotoxicity with a 50 mg/m² dose.

Patients achieving CR after the 12-week induction treatment were then randomized to receive either MCT for 2 years or RT to the areas of previous tumor involvement. If partial remission (PR) was attained in patients with solitary pulmonary metastases, surgical resections of residual tumor were performed followed by MCT. In the other patients with PR, the above induction chemotherapy was repeated and patients with CR after this second induction treatment were then randomized to receive either MCT or RT, whereas patients with persisting PR were given MCT. Patients with a <50% response, no change, or progressive disease were dropped from the study as treatment failures.

MCT consisted of cyclohexyl chlorethyl nitrosourea (CCNU) (100 mg/m²) every 8 weeks plus alternating weekly VBL (7 mg/m²) and oral methotrexate (20 mg/m²) (Fig. 1).

In a retrospective analysis, patients were subdivided according to the tumor burden into patients with minimal disease and patients with advanced disease. The following

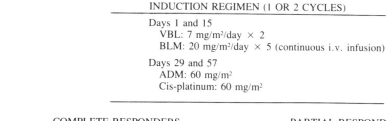

INDUCTION REGIMEN (1 OR 2 CYCLES)

Days 1 and 15
  VBL: 7 mg/m²/day × 2
  BLM: 20 mg/m²/day × 5 (continuous i.v. infusion)

Days 29 and 57
  ADM: 60 mg/m²
  Cis-platinum: 60 mg/m²

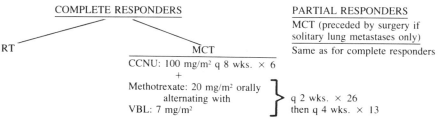

COMPLETE RESPONDERS

RT   MCT

CCNU: 100 mg/m² q 8 wks. × 6
  +
Methotrexate: 20 mg/m² orally
  alternating with
VBL: 7 mg/m²   q 2 wks. × 26
                      then q 4 wks. × 13

PARTIAL RESPONDERS

MCT (preceded by surgery if solitary lung metastases only)
Same as for complete responders

FIG. 1.   Induction and maintenance schedules for metastatic testicular cancer.

patients were evaluated as having minimal disease: by lung metastases, if they had less than 10 metastases and all smaller than 3 cm; by abdominal disease, if in the lymphangiogram none of the positive lymph nodes were bigger than 3 cm and if there was no deviation of the ureters and no distortion of the vena cava. All other patients were considered to have advanced disease. Those criteria were not used to stratify patients before the randomization.

CR was defined as complete disappearance of all measurable and nonmeasurable tumor parameters as well as a return to normal of tumor markers such as α-fetoprotein and human chorionic gonadotropin, if these were initially elevated. A PR indicated a reduction of >50% in the product of two perpendicular tumor diameters.

Initial drug doses were reduced by 25% if the patient had undergone extensive RT, especially to the abdominal and pelvic regions, within 2 months of starting treatment. If no undue toxicity was observed during the first cycle of BLM and VBL, the doses were increased to 100%. Normal renal function (with a BUN level <30 mg/dl or a serum creatinine level <1.8 mg/dl) was mandatory for BLM or cis-platinum administration. The doses of subsequent courses of treatment were reduced by 25% for the following reasons: persisting leukopenia (between 3,000 and 4,000 cells/mm^3) or thrombocytopenia (between 90,000 and 120,000 cells/mm^3), a leukocyte nadir <1,000/mm^3 or a platelet nadir <20,000/mm^3, persisting mucositis, severe obstipation with symptoms of ileus, or fever >39°C not controlled with prednisone. MCT doses were reduced by 50% for leukocyte counts between 2,500 and 4,000/mm^3 or platelet counts between 50,000 and 100,000/mm^3. Therapy was withheld if lower values or persisting mucositis occurred.

Megavoltage RT was applied to all known areas of tumor involvement at the start of the study. The fields were to extend 4 cm beyond the known tumor area wherever possible. A dose of 4,000 rads given over 4 to 5 weeks for field areas <300 cm^2 was planned. For field areas >300 cm^2, the dose was reduced to 3,000 rads. The total dose to the kidneys was not to exceed 1,700 rads over 4 weeks, and the total dose to the liver was limited to 2,500 rads. If the irradiated lung volume was ≤30% of the total lung volume, a midline dose of 2,500 rads was given with daily doses of 180 to 200 rads. For irradiated volumes up to 50% of the total lung volume, the dose was 1,800 rads with daily doses of 150 to 160 rads. For irradiated volumes >50% of the total lung volume, the dose was 1,500 rads with 100-rad daily doses.

RESULTS

As of February 1980, 129 patients were entered in the study. Of these, 27 were not evaluable. Twelve had not yet completed their first induction cycle. Gross protocol violations with regard to treatment sequence, timing, or randomization occurred in 10. Two patients were ineligible because no measurable tumor was present, and another developed an acute glomerulonephritis so that cis-platinum could not be given.

Of the 102 evaluable patients, there were 18 (18%) patients with PR. The median duration of PR was only 3.1 months (range, 0.3 to 8.3 months). The median survival was 7 months (range, 0.8 to 22 months). There were 63 (62%) patients with CR; 2 of these resulted from resection of a residual lung lesion. Only 15 (23%) of the patients with CR relapsed, including the 2 patients who had undergone surgical resection of residual lung metastases. Both of these tumors contained choriocarcinoma components, and 1 patient had refused MCT.

After randomization, 30 patients with CR received MCT and 22 with CR were irradiated. Nine relapses have occurred in the MCT group between 2 and 13 months. In the RT group, there have been only 6 relapses between 4 and 10 months. After a mean observation of more than 2 years, the median remission duration has yet to be reached in both groups (MCT and RT).

Toxicity encountered during the induction chemotherapy phase of treatment was moderately severe. It manifested itself mainly in the form of hematologic toxicity following the BLM/VBL cycles and was less severe with ADM/cis-platinum (Table 1). Other forms of toxicity included an almost universal alopecia, BLM-induced fever (70%), obstipation with abdominal pain, and symptoms of ileus resulting from BLM/VBL treatment were encountered in about 50% of the courses and were considered moderately severe in 20%. Mucositis was frequent with BLM/VBL (40%) and was moderate to very severe in 15% of the cases. Nausea and vomiting were recorded in about ⅓ of the BLM/VBL courses. This form of toxicity was almost universal with ADM/cis-platinum.

Renal toxicity with cis-platinum was not a problem with the modes of administration used in this study. Elevated BUN and/or serum creatinine values were seen in 7% of the courses. Only 3 patients had persisting serum creatinine values between 1.7 and 2.0 mg/dl. Myalgia and arthralgia were common with BLM/VBL. Only 1 case of BLM-induced lung toxicity has been documented; it was not fatal. Two drug-related deaths occurred during induction treatment. The first patient, with extensive abdominal tumor masses, underwent laparotomy on day 9 of treatment for intestinal obstruction. Three days after surgery, the peripheral granulocyte count was 36/mm^3. By day 16, the leukocyte count had recovered to 9,900/mm^3, and,

TABLE 1. *Hematologic toxicity during induction phase*

	Leukocyte count (cells × 10³/mm³)		Platelet count (cells × 10³/mm³)	Hemoglobin level (g/100 ml)	
	1.0–1.9	<1.0	<50.0	3–4	>4
BLM/VBL (total = 89 courses)	29	35	18	17	10
ADM/cis-platinum (total = 82 courses)	14	3	2		
MCT (total = 24 courses)	14	0	1	NE[a]	NE

[a]NE = Not evaluated.

in violation of the protocol, another full dose of BLM/VBL was given. This resulted in wound dehiscence, fecal peritonitis, agranulocytosis, sepsis, and death on day 25. The second death occurred in a patient with initially normal serum creatinine values (0.7 to 1.2 mg/dl). Again, despite a leukocyte nadir of $500/mm^3$ during the first BLM/VBL course, full doses of these drugs were repeated. On day 3 of this second course, the serum creatinine value was 2.0 mg/dl and continuously rose to 95 mg/dl. The leukocyte count subsequently fell to $90/mm^3$ with 0 granulocytes, and the patient died on day 26 of the study with an *Escherichia coli* sepsis. The cause of the renal insufficiency which was present before the patient became septic and certainly contributed to the fatal outcome is not entirely clear. It may have resulted from a 5-day gentamicin treatment (240 mg given daily on days 9 to 13).

DISCUSSION

The first goal of this study, to attain a high CR rate with induction chemotherapy, was achieved (62%). Disregarded in these results are at least two CR in the non-evaluable group. One had to be dropped from the study because of an acute glomerulonephritis which made cis-platinum treatment impossible. Another never received RT as per randomization.

The two toxic deaths occurred in the face of frank protocol violations. They may have been avoided by strict adherence to the protocol stipulations of dose reduction. This lethal toxicity rate of 2% compares well to the 6.4% (3 of 47 patients), lethal toxicity rate reported in the only other study of this size to date with a CR rate >50% with chemotherapy alone (3).

TABLE 2. *Patient characteristics: Histology and therapeutic results*

	Median age (yr)	Histology	
		Embryonal cell (%)	Choriocarcinoma (%)
All patients	28	40	14.5
Complete responders	29	60	11.4
Complete responders: MCT	28.5	60	5
Complete responders: RT	24	60	20

TABLE 3. *Tumor burden and therapeutic results*

	Minimal disease No. of patients	Advanced disease No. of patients
Total	37 (41%)	54 (59%)
CR	35 (95%)	19 (35%)
CR relapse	7 (20%)	8 (42%)
Alive	31 (84%)	17 (31%)

Unexpected toxicity in the RT arm of this study was not encountered despite the intensive chemotherapy pretreatment. Even 10 total lung irradiations following BLM doses of up to 700 mg (270 to 700 mg) have been tolerated to date. It appears, therefore, that RT is of definite value for the consolidation of CR induced by chemotherapy in this disease. Whether it is superior to MCT still remains to be seen.

Failure to achieve long-term remission in our 2 patients undergoing surgical resection of residual pulmonary disease is disappointing. It does not correlate with our own previous experience or that of Einhorn and Donohue (3). One patient with a survival of only 10 months had refused MCT; the other is alive with disease at 16 months. Surgery was probably performed too early in these patients and should have been preceded by a second course of induction therapy.

A comparison of the patient characteristics in the RT- and MCT-treated groups (Table 2) shows the RT patients to be slightly younger. Twenty percent of these had choriocarcinomatous components in their tumors, and there was abdominal disease present in almost 50%. Table 2 also suggests that patients with tumors of the embryonal cell type, with or without seminoma, but lacking other histologic tissue types, were more likely to undergo CR with induction chemotherapy than patients with other forms or mixed tumors. There were 40% such "pure" embryonal cell tumors in the entire patient population, 60% in those attaining CR, and 16% (only 4 in 25 patients) not attaining CR. This last difference for the nonresponders is statistically significant ($p = 0.003$).

As can be seen from Table 3, there is a clear-cut correlation between the initial tumor burden and the therapeutic outcome. The CR rate for patients with minimal disease is 95%, whereas the CR rate for patients with advanced disease is only 35% ($p < 0.01$). Also, regarding the relapses after having achieved CR, there is a significant difference between the two categories of patients: only ⅕ of the CR

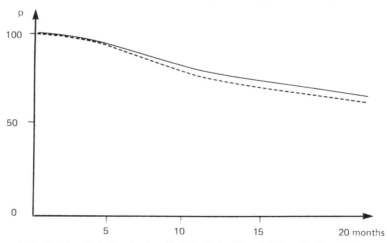

FIG. 2. Survival of patients with CR. *Dotted line*, MCT; *solid line*, RT.

patients with minimal disease relapsed, whereas almost 50% of the patients with advanced disease relapsed. Studies correlating tumor burden and histologic type are still ongoing: from a preliminary analysis of the study, it seems that the tumor burden is of greater importance than the histologic type as a prognostic determinant for the therapeutic outcome. These very important data have still to be ascertained by further analysis, however.

A definite evaluation of remission duration and survival is not yet possible, since most patients in CR remain free of tumor and are still living (Fig. 2). In view of the results achieved, we feel that the toxicity encountered with this treatment regimen is acceptable. Lethal toxicity may well be avoidable if strict precautions for dose adjustment and patient and laboratory controls are followed. The risk and discomfort as well as the expenditure of time and effort seem to be adequately compensated for in terms of survival and possible cure in this group of young patients.

For the time being, we can therefore confirm the findings of other studies concerning the therapeutic results achieved with dichlorodiammineplatinum-containing regimens (3). It is, however, possible that patients presenting with advanced disease in the future will require a treatment even more aggressive than that used in our study.

REFERENCES

1. Blum, R. H., Carter, S. K., and Agre, K. (1973): A clinical review of bleomycin—a new antineoplastic agent. *Cancer*, 31:903–914.
2. Cvitkovic, E., Hayes, D., and Golbey, R. (1976): Primary combination chemotherapy (VAB III) for metastatic or unresectable germ cell tumors. *Proc. Am. Assoc. Cancer Res. and ASCO*, 17:296.
3. Einhorn, L. H., and Donohue, J. (1977): Cis-diamminedichloroplatinum, vinblastine, and bleomycin combination chemotherapy in disseminated testicular cancer. *Ann. Intern. Med.*, 87:293–298.
4. Higby, D. J., Wallace, H. J., Jr., and Holland, J. F. (1973): Cis-diamminedichloroplatinum (NSC-119875): A phase I study. *Cancer Chemother. Rep.*, 57:459–463.
5. Mackenzie, A. R. (1966): Chemotherapy of metastatic testis cancer: Results in 154 patients. *Cancer*, 19:1,369–1,376.
6. Samuels, M. L., Holoye, P. Y., and Johnson, D. E. (1975): Bleomycin combination chemotherapy in the management of testicular neoplasia. *Cancer*, 36:318–325.
7. Samuels, M. L., and Howe, C. D. (1970): Vinblastine in the management of testicular cancer. *Cancer*, 25:1,009–1,017.
8. Sonntag, R. W., Brunner, K. W., Batz, K., and Ryssel, H. J. (1975): Treatment of metastatic testicular carcinoma with bleomycin (NSC-125066) used alone or in combination with CCNU (NSC-79037). *Cancer Chemother. Rep.*, 59:429–431.
9. Vogl, S., Ohnuma, T., Perloff, M., and Holland, J. F. (1976): Combination chemotherapy with adriamycin and cis-diamminedichloroplatinum in patients with neoplastic diseases. *Cancer*, 38:21–26.

New Approaches in Cancer Therapy,
edited by H. Cortés Funes and M. Rozencweig.
Raven Press, New York © 1982.

Cisplatin, Vinblastine, and Bleomycin Combination Chemotherapy for Advanced Germ Cell Tumors

H. Cortés Funes, O. Leiva, C. Mendiola, M. Mendez, and A. Moyano

Hospital "1º de Octubre," Madrid, Spain

Germ cell tumors have a common histopathologic denominator. They arise mainly in the gonads, more frequently in the testicle than the ovary, but can be located in extragonadal sites. These tumors are among the most perplexing and embryologically intriguing entities in clinical oncology. In contrast to other solid tumors, the introduction of chemotherapy has dramatically prolonged survival in patients with disseminated disease. This improvement in survival is related in part to the multidisciplinary approach: urologists, radiotherapists, surgeons, and medical oncologists are involved in the care of such patients.

The most representative group among these malignancies is the primary testicular germ cell tumor. Testicular tumors occur in 1 to 2% of cancers in male patients. They rank as the leading cause of death in the 25- to 44-year-old age group (14), with an estimated 2,500 new cases per year in the U.S. This cancer constitutes the fourth most common genitourinary tumor. The overall incidence of testicular tumors in Europe has been reported as 2 to 2.5 per 100,000 male subjects per year (18). When first seen, 35% of the patients have either lymphatic dissemination or distant metastases. Primary treatment increases the number of patients with testicular cancer who require chemotherapy to approximately 50%.

Combination chemotherapy for advanced testicular cancer has been used since 1960 when Li et al. introduced the combination of actinomycin-D (ACD), chlorambucil (CLB), and methotrexate (MTX), obtaining a 50 to 70% response rate with 10 to 20% complete remission (13). Since that time, other researchers have reported similar results (1,15) and other new agents have been incorporated in different combinations with marginally improved results. Most notably, these studies substantiated that complete remissions, as well as permanent cures, could be obtained in disseminated testicular cancer (1,12,15,22). The vast majority of relapses occurs within 2 years of initiation of chemotherapy.

Since 1970, the results of chemotherapy in advanced testicular tumors have improved considerably. Samuels et al. doubled the complete response rate using a combination of vinblastine (VBL) and bleomycin (BLM) (23,24). At that time, phase I studies of cisplatin (DDP) done by Higby et al. (9) demonstrated considerable single-agent activity against testicular carcinoma. Subsequently, a combination of DDP with the original Samuels' combination of VBL and BLM (PVB) was developed at Indiana University by Einhorn and Donahue, who reported a 74% complete remission rate and 26% partial remission rate in 50 patients with disseminated testicular cancer (5). Long-term follow-up of these patients demonstrated that less than 10% of complete responders relapsed. This indicates that more than 65% of the original patients with advanced disease were in remission for more than 5 years, thus confirming complete eradication of disease (6). Other investigators have confirmed this data with different (8) or similar combinations (20,21,25; Sonntag et al., *this volume*).

Since 1974, we have been using this original Einhorn combination of PVB in a group of patients with advanced resistant germ cell tumors. The results of the treatment in 66 patients are analyzed in this chapter.

MATERIAL AND METHODS

Sixty-six fully evaluable patients who presented with histologically confirmed germ cell primary tumor of the testis, ovary, and extragonadal localization in advanced stage not previously treated, or recurrent after surgery, radiotherapy, or chemotherapy were entered in this study between October 1976 and July 1980. Patients with seminomas were ineligible during the first part of the study, but due to the high response rate obtained with this regimen, the protocol was expanded to include primary advanced and/or recurrent seminomas. All patients had measurable metastatic disease and were not refractory to any of the study agents. Patients who died within 3 weeks of initiation of chemotherapy were considered inevaluable.

Pretreatment evaluation included a complete history and examination, performance status, hemoglobin, white blood cell with differential and platelet count, clinical chemistry profile (SMA-12), creatinine clearance, and urinalysis. Alphafetoprotein (AFP) and beta-subunit of human chorionic gonadotropin (b-HCG) were done at the beginning of the study only in complete responders to confirm their status. Afterwards, when the technique was introduced routinely in our hospital, it was done before and after treatment. Biologic markers were used in all patients during the follow-up period. Other studies were chest X-ray, bone scintigraphy, and computerized tomography (CT) thoracoabdominal scan.

All measurable tumor lesions were documented, and positive studies were repeated after three cycles of treatment to establish the type of remission obtained, indicating subsequent treatment.

Patients were treated with the PVB combination in two different schedules, which were evaluated independently. The first 19 patients (Table 1) received DDP for 5 consecutive days (days 2 to 6) at a dosage of 20 mg/m² body surface area. Medication was administered as a 1-hr. i.v. infusion with 12 hr of pre- and posthydration with 3,000 cc in 5% dextrose in normal saline. Diuresis was induced with 25 g of mannitol given before and after dosage. VBL was administered at 6 mg/m² (3

TABLE 1. *Treatment scheme for first series of patients*

DDP: 20 mg/m^2, i.v., days 2–6, every 3 weeks for 1 year
VBL: 3 mg/m^2, i.v., days 1 and 2, every 3 weeks for 1 year
BLM: 30 U, i.v. weekly 12 times and in each cycle (day 2)
     afterwards

TABLE 2. *Treatment scheme for second series of patients*

Induction
  DDP: 100 mg/m^2, i.v., day 2
  VBL: 6 mg/m^2, i.v., days 1 and 2
  BLM: 30 u, i.v. continuous infusion, days 2–6
three times every 3–4 weeks
Maintenance
  Complete remission: DDP and VBL, same dosage for six cycles
  Partial remission: DDP and VBL at same dosage adding a third active drug alternating
    each cycle with the following sequence: ACD: 1 mg/m^2, i.v. (4th cycle); CTX: 600
    mg/m^2, i.v. (5th cycle); and ADM: 45 mg/m^2, i.v. (6th cycle); all on day 2.

mg/m^2 each day). Both drugs were repeated every 3 weeks for 1 year or until relapse. BLM was given weekly, by i.v. push starting on day 2, for the first 12 weeks and then every 3 weeks for 1 year or until relapse.

The second series of 47 patients received the same PVB regimen administered in combination with other agents on a modified dosage schedule whenever complete response was not achieved after three cycles. In the second schedule (Table 2), DDP was given at a dosage of 100 mg/m^2 of body surface area in 1 day (day 2) with the same hydration and mannitol-induced diuresis regimen as in the first schedule. In both groups of patients, intake and output of fluids and electrolytes were monitored and replaced as needed after measurements of urine output and emesis. Dosage of VBL was doubled, given 12 mg/m^2 in 2 days (days 1 and 2), at the beginning of prehydration and repeated at 12-hr intervals. BLM was administered at 30 u dissolved in 1,000 cc of 5% dextrose in normal saline in continuous 24-hr daily infusions for 5 consecutive days, immediately after the postDDP hydration. The entire cycle was repeated on day 26 if the patient had recovered from hematologic and renal toxicity.

Patients achieving a complete response after three cycles continued on treatment with DDP and VBL at the same dosage for nine more cycles. Patients achieving only partial response after three cycles of PVB were continued on chemotherapy with DDP and VBL at the same dosage while BLM was replaced by a rotation of a third active drug—cyclophosphamide (CTX), ACD, or adriamycin (ADM) (Table 2). Response was reevaluated after this treatment and surgery for residual tumors was considered for those patients still in partial remission. Those patients who achieved complete response following the second cycle series were maintained on the same therapeutic schedule with DDP and VBL for six more cycles.

Patient characteristics are detailed in Table 3. There were 57 males and 9 females. Primary disease was in testicle (43 patients), ovary (6 patients), and extragonadal tumors (14 mediastinal, 2 retroperitoneal, and 1 sacrococcygeal). In the first series of patients, 78.9% had been previously treated with chemotherapy, radiotherapy, or both. Only 31.2% of the patients in the second series had received prior therapy. Median follow-up of patients was 32+ months with a range from 10+ to 54+ months, and somewhat longer in the first group of patients.

GONADAL TUMORS

This group was comprised of 49 patients: 6 with ovarian and 43 with testicular disease. Patient characteristics are detailed in Table 4 and 5.

The ovarian tumor group was comprised of 6 fully evaluable patients. All had advanced disease, and all except 1 were treated with the second regimen. Median follow-up was 21.8 months (range, from 6 to 50+ months). Histologic types were 2 teratomas, 2 disgerminomas, 1 yolk sac, and 1 embryonal carcinoma. Five patients had been previously treated with chemotherapy and/or radiotherapy. All patients achieved complete remission. There was only 1 relapse at the 6th month, not responding to other chemotherapy, who died soon after from progression of disease.

TABLE 3. *Germ cell tumors—Patient characteristics*

	1st Series	2nd Series	Total
Number	19	47	66
Male	18	39	57
Female	1	8	9
Testicular	17	26	43
Ovary	1	5	6
Extragonadal	1	16	17
Prior chemotherapy	10	5	15
Prior radiotherapy	—	8	8
Both	5	2	7
Median follow-up, months (range)	42+(30+,54+)	20+(10+,31+)	32+(10+,54+)

TABLE 4. *Ovarian tumors*

N	Age	Histology	Prior Rx	Stage	Response	Follow-up
1	24	Embryonal	CT	II (A)	CR	50+ mo. NED
2	13	Disgerminoma	—	II (A)	CR	23+ mo. NED
3	26	Teratoma	CT	II (A)	CR	22+ mo. NED
4	19	Yolk sac	RT–CT	III (P–A)	CR	22+ mo. NED
5	21	Disgerminoma	RT	III (P–A)	CR	6+ mo., relapse–died
6	23	Teratoma/yolk sac	CT	III (P–A)	CR	18+ mo. NED

Abbreviations: A, advanced abdominal; P, advanced pulmonary; CR, complete response; NED, no evidence of disease.

TABLE 5. *Testicular tumors—Patient characteristics*

Treatment	1st Series		2nd Series		Total	
Number	17		26		43	
Age (median)	28.5		30.7		29.6	
Prior therapy	14	(82.6%)	15	(57.6%)	29	
Chemotherapy	5		4		9	
Radiotherapy	—		8		8	
Chemotherapy and radiotherapy	9		3		12	
None	3		11		14	
Follow-up, months (range)	40	(28–52+)	18+	(8–29+)	30+	(8–52+)

The other 5 patients are free of disease with a follow-up period ranging from 18+ to 50+ months.

The testicular tumor group included 43 patients. Median age was 29.6 years (range, from 19 to 42 years). Median follow-up of patients was 30+ months with a range from 8 to 52+ months, and somewhat longer in the group of patients in the first regimen. Patient responses to the PVB schedule reported in the two different series were evaluated separately in order to obtain unified treatment results.

In the first series of 17 patients, there were 6 complete remissions (35.3%) and 9 partial remissions (59.9%), giving an overall response rate of 88.2%. There was 1 death in a patient with complete remission without relapse at the 11th month, attributed to gastrointestinal bleeding induced by a peptic ulcer. There were no relapses in the remaining from 28+ to 52+ months. Three of the 6 complete remissions had had no previous treatment, and the other 3 had received short-term courses of the Li regimen (13) before PVB treatment.

All partial responders and the 2 nonresponders had been previously treated. All complete responders continued treatment for a 1-year period. BLM was discontinued in 2 patients at a total dosage of 560 and 430 U for asymptomatic lung function reduction. The other 3 patients received a total BLM dosage of 630, 750, and 760 U with no toxicity. Total cumulative dosage of DDP in these series was over 1,000 mg.

In the second series of 26 evaluable patients, 19 (73%) patients achieved complete response. Three of these complete responses were obtained following resection of residual nonmalignant tissue in patients originally classified as partial responders. Of the remaining 7 patients, partial response was reported in 4 and no response in the last 3. Of these, 2 died after the second treatment course, and the last patient died due to disease progression after the third course. In all cases, therapy had been administered for very advanced tumors in heavily pretreated patients with a low performance status. Of the 19 complete responders, 10 had had no prior therapy, whereas the remaining 9 had received chemotherapy only. Three of these 9 patients had been on the Li regimen (13), 4 on ADM-based combinations, and the last 2 patients had received light doses of VBL and BLM but were considered eligible for entry into this study.

Administration of CTX, ACD, and ADM in rotation to patients who had not achieved complete remission following the first three PVB courses produced no change in these patients. Administration of the seventh treatment cycle combining all active drugs to 2 patients who had achieved partial response produced no positive therapeutic results but considerable toxicity.

Three complete responders relapsed at 6, 9, and 11 months, respectively. In 2 of these patients, there was metastatic brain involvement. Both underwent surgery followed by brain irradiation. Another resection was performed in 1 of these 2 patients who developed a second cerebral metastasis undetected by the previous CT scan and is free of disease 6 months after this last surgery. The other patient with brain metastasis had another relapse at the abdominal level and had a new response with the second-line combination of DDP, VP-16, and ADM.

Median follow-up for this second series of patients was 18+ months. The 16 complete responders without relapse have a follow-up period ranging from 8 to 29+ months. There were no relapses after 12 months in both series of patients. At the present time, all 5 patients still alive in the first series and 14 out of 16 patients in the second series have been in complete remission for a period of up to 12 months.

Four patients underwent surgery and remained in partial remission after six cycles of the second chemotherapeutic regimen.

Two of the 3 patients who underwent thoracotomy had no malignant tissue upon resection. The 3rd patient had two lesions that had metastasized to the lung from an embryonal carcinoma. The first lesion was completely necrotic. A partial resection was done of the second lesion and it was fixed to the posterior thoracic wall. The tissue of this second metastatic lesion was similar to the first, containing necrotic material and a few signs of malignant embryonal carcinoma cells. This patient died of disseminated lung disease 25 months after beginning treatment.

The remaining patient achieved a complete response after the resection of a retroperitoneal residual mass which was a mature teratoma with no malignant elements. We have observed transformation of malignant teratomas into benign teratomas after aggressive chemotherapy with other combinations. This finding has been published by several authors (10,11,17,26).

There was no correlation between response and pathology. Response rate had a direct relationship to the extent of the disease.

EXTRAGONADAL TUMORS

Extragonadal tumors included 17 patients with the following localizations: 2 retroperitoneal, 1 sacrococcygeal, and 14 mediastinal. Patient characteristics of the group are detailed in Table 6. There were 14 males and 3 females with a median age of 29 years (range, 2 to 50). Four patients had embryonal carcinomas, 4 had malignant teratomas, 1 had choriocarcinoma, 4 had pure seminomas, and the other 4 had mixed tumors.

A 24-year-old woman with primary mediastinal choriocarcinoma was excluded from the evaluation. The autopsy confirmed the diagnosis of mediastinal germ cell

TABLE 6. *Extragonadal germ cell tumors*

Sex	Primary (histology)	Prior therapy	Extension	Response	Duration and evolution
M	MED—mixed	No	Mediastinum—liver	PR	12 Mo—Died tumor progression
M	MED—seminoma	No	Mediastinum—lung	CR	31 + Mo—NED
M	MED—embryonal	No	Mediastinum	CR	31 + Mo—NED
M	MED—mixed	No	Mediastinum—liver	NR	3 Mo—Died tumor progression
M	MED—seminoma	MTX–ACD CLB–RT	Mediastinum—lung	CR	30 + Mo—NED
M	MED—embryonal	MTX–ACD–CLB	Mediastinum	CR	11 Mo—Died drug toxicity
F	MED—chorroca	No	Mediastinum—pleura	NE	Died tumor progression
M	MED—seminoma	No	Mediastinum—pericardium	CR	15 + Mo—NED, corrobated by biopsy
F	MED—embryonal	No	Mediastinum—cervical nodes	PR	7 Mo—No response to RT and 2nd PR to VP-16-DDP-ADM, alive in PR
M	MED—mixed	ADM–CTX	Mediastinum—cervical nodes	PR	6 Mo—RT; Died tumor progression
M	MED—seminoma	No	Mediastinum	CR	10 Mo—Relapse, PR with RT, relapse and in CR with VP-16-DDP-ADM
M	MED—embryonal	No	Mediastinum—lung—pleura	NR	3 Mo—Died tumor progression
M	MED—teratoma	No	Mediastinum—lung	PR	2 Mo—RT—No response—Died by tumor progression 12 mo after
M	MED—teratoma	No	Mediastinum—lung—liver	NR	2 Mo—Died tumor progression
M	ABD—mixed	No	Retroperitoneum—liver—inguinal nodes	PR	3 Mo—Died tumor progression
F	Sacroc. teratoma	No	Sacrococcygeal—abdomen	CR	18 + Mo—NED
M	ABD—mixed	No	Retroperitoneum—liver	PR	8 Mo—Died tumor progression

Abbreviations: PR, partial remission; CR, complete remission; NR, no response; NE, nonevaluable; NED, no evidence of disease.

tumor. Only 3 patients had received prior treatment, 2 with chemotherapy and the other with radiotherapy and chemotherapy.

The 2 retroperitoneal patients had a partial response to the second regimen and died from progression of disease at 6 and 9 months. A 2-year-old girl with sacrococcygeal tumor achieved a complete remission after three cycles of PVB and is still free of disease with a follow-up of 18 + months.

Of the 13 mediastinal patients evaluated for response to chemotherapy (Table 7), 6 patients (46.1%) achieved a complete remission. Four other patients (30.7%) obtained a partial remission for an overall response rate of 76.9%. All patients with seminomas achieved complete remission; 1 of them relapsed 1 month after discontinuing chemotherapy. This patient had had no previous treatment and was treated with radiation therapy, obtaining a new remission, for a short period of time; immediately after the end of radiotherapy, the patient developed lung metastasis and bilateral pleural effusion. A new complete remission was obtained with a second-line chemotherapy regimen, mentioned before, which included DDP, VP-16-213, and ADM. The other 3 seminoma patients were not treated primarily with radiotherapy because of the extent of the tumor with lung infiltration. They are in complete remission for a period of 31 +, 30 +, and 15 + months, respectively. Two other patients with primary embryonal carcinoma of the mediastinum also obtained a complete response. One died from drug toxicity at 11 months and the other remained free of disease for 31 + months.

As mentioned before, 4 of the 13 mediastinal patients achieved a partial remission of their disease ranging from 2 to 12 months. One of these patients, with a mixed embryonal and choriocarcinoma with documented liver metastasis, achieved a good partial response for 4 months. The other 3 partial responders were treated with radiotherapy without response, with 2 of them dying at 7 and 9 months. The 3rd partial responder had a minor response to radiation therapy, but developed bilateral lung metastasis. At the present time, this patient is alive and responding to a DDP, VP-16, and ADM combination. Three other patients had no response to chemotherapy and died from tumor progression in a period of 4 months.

TOXICITY

Toxicity was also evaluated separately in both series of all patient groups and is detailed in Table 8. Toxicity was mild in the first series and more intensive in the second one. This toxicity was mainly due to DDP, which produced nausea and vomiting in all patients when administered as an infusion for 5 days to patients in the first series and for 1 day only to patients in the second series.

It is important to mention that nephrotoxicity was very low in both series of patients (13%) with no acute renal failure. Only 9 patients had serum creatinine levels up to 2 mg% before treatment: 8 patients in the first series and 1 in the second. It is also important to remember that, in both regimens, DDP was given for a long period of time, achieving a cumulative dosage of approximately 1,000 mg in each case. Following administration of a cumulative dose of up to 500 mg

TABLE 7. *Mediastinal germ cell tumors—*
Patient characteristics

Number	14
Evaluable	13
Male/female	11/2
Age (range)	31.3 (21–50)
Prior CT or RT	3
Embryonal carcinomas	4
Teratomas	2
Seminomas	4
Mixed	3

TABLE 8. *Mediastinal germ cell tumors: Responses*

Complete remission	6/13 (46.1%)
Partial remission	4/13 (30.7%)
Global response	10/13 (76.9%)
Relapses after CR	1 (7.7%)
Alive NED	4 (31 +,31 +,30 +,15 + months)

TABLE 9. *Toxicity*

	1st Series	2nd Series	Total	(%)
Nausea and vomiting	19	48	67	(100)
Reduction in renal function (creatinine clearance <50 ml/min and/or serum creatinine ≥2 mg%)	8	1	9	(13)
WBC ≤2,000/mm³	6	30	36	(54)
Platelets ≤100,000/mm³	—	18	18	(27)
Fever (noninfectious)	4	29	33	(49)
Mucositis	—	14	14	(21)
Alopecia	3	28	31	(46)
Dermatitis	1	14	15	(22)
Abdominal pain	—	11	11	(16)
Neurotoxicity (paresthesias and EMG alterations[a] and/ or tinnitus)	4	12	16	(24)
Drug-related deaths	2	1	3	(4)

[a]EMG studies done in 11 patients.

of DDP, levels of creatinine clearance tended to fall. These reduced levels recovered with time. The correlation between renal toxicity and dosage has been discussed in other publications (19).

Mild hypokalemia and hypomagnesemia were occasionally seen without clinical manifestation. This was due to alterations in electrolyte balance occurring during the posthydration period. We found important electrophysiologic alterations in all patients studied. These patients had mild paresthesias and deep tendon reflex loss.

This clinical picture was attributed to a peripheral neuropathy produced by high cumulative doses of DDP. A sural biopsy was performed in 2 patients who presented with axon demyelination with neurofibril disruption. This has been reported in another study (16). Tinnitus was observed by several patients but had no clinical significance.

Leukopenia was seen frequently in the second group of patients (54%) and was considered severe in some cases. Nadir usually occurred between day 7 and 14 and was about 1,000/mm³. Only 2 patients were hospitalized with granulocytopenic fever. They were treated successfully with antibiotics. Thrombocytopenia, observed in 27% of the patients in the second series, was less marked. No patient suffered bleeding episodes or required platelet transfusions. All complaints of abdominal pain were attributed to the higher doses of VBL used in the second series of patients.

BLM produced noninfectious fever and chills, dermatitis, and alopecia. However, these reactions were not serious and did not require discontinuation of medication. Pulmonary function was altered in 2 patients who had received a cumulative dosage of 400 U BLM.

There were 3 drug-related deaths, 2 in the first series and 1 in the second. As previously stated, 1 testicular patient died following an episode of gastric bleeding. The 2nd patient also had a testicular tumor; serious toxicity developed following administration of the third PVB cycle and he expired from a massive pulmonary embolism. At autopsy, this patient was found to be in complete remission. The 3rd drug-related death was due to BLM lung syndrome in a patient with a mediastinal embryonal carcinoma. This patient died of acute respiratory failure and the autopsy showed no evidence of tumor.

DISCUSSION

As we mentioned at the beginning of this chapter, germ cell tumors are different diseases with a common embryologic origin and pathologic appearance. They are located most frequently in the testicle or ovary, but can also be primarily located in extragonadal sites.

Both groups of tumors, gonadal and extragonadal, have the same sensitivity to the different therapeutic modalities. In advanced stages, chemotherapy is indicated. The introduction of new chemotherapy regimens with DDP has achieved a high complete response rate in testicular tumors and, more or less, the same results in ovary and extragonadal tumors. Some authors claim (21) that those therapeutic results obtained with chemotherapy in gonadal tumors are different from those in extragonadal tumors, as the latter are less responsive.

Extragonadal germ cell tumors are a definite clinicopathologic entity. They occur mainly in young males with a retroperitoneal or anterior mediastinal mass and an initial pathologic diagnosis of "neoplasm primary unknown" (4). Modern aggressive combination chemotherapy with DDP has improved the median survival and potential cure rate in these patients (7).

Extragonadal patients included 14 primary mediastinal, 2 retroperitoneal, and 1 sacrococcygeal tumor. Only partial remissions of short duration were obtained in retroperitoneal primary tumors. The patient with sacrococcygeal germ cell tumor achieved complete remission and remains free of disease 18 + months after diagnosis. The mediastinal tumors in our series were less responsive than testicular tumors, with a global response rate of 76.9% and only 46% in complete remission. There was 1 relapse who then achieved a new complete response with VP-16 combination chemotherapy. One patient in complete remission died from drug toxicity due to BLM lung syndrome. The remaining 4 patients originally in complete remission remained free of disease with a follow-up period ranging from 15 + to 31 + months.

With the primary mediastinal germ cell tumors, it is important to note that there are some differences in therapy and probably in response rates between the different histologies. Our series included 4 seminomas, 3 of which were not candidates to receive radiotherapy because of the extent of disease. The 3rd one was treated with chemotherapy on the basis of the good results obtained with the other tumors. This last patient relapsed after discontinuing chemotherapy and achieved a new remission of short duration with radiotherapy, because of developing lung metastasis and malignant pleural effusion. Another complete response was obtained with VP-16-213, DDP, and ADM, a combination that demonstrates considerable activity against this type of tumor.

The rest of the primary mediastinal seminoma patients continued free of disease with a follow-up range from 15 + to 31 + months. The other 2 complete responders had embryonal carcinomas; 1 is free of disease after 31 + months and the other died, without tumor, due to drug toxicity at 11 months. All partial responders, except 1, died from tumor progression in a relatively short period of time. Radiation therapy has no role in these resistant patients.

The ovarian germ cell tumors responded in exactly the same way as testicular tumors and should be treated with the same procedures. Our response rate for testicular tumor was 35% in the first group of 17 heavily pretreated patients. We reconsidered the treatment and then developed a new PVB basis from our experience in the first series of patients, using a full dosage of VBL and a few other modifications mentioned before. With this new regimen we were able to reproduce Einhorn's 73% initial complete remissions in the second series of 26 patients.

Although the series are not comparable, the following is evident: the effectiveness of DDP is demonstrated, but the role of VBL at high dose (6 mg/m^2 or 3 mg/kg) is not confirmed. Einhorn also felt that no therapeutic benefit could be achieved by increasing these dose levels (6).

In future studies, it will be our goal to identify the 30% of initially resistant patients, as well as the 10 to 15% who will later relapse. This information will enable us to identify the reason for such resistance (most probably related to prognostic factors) in the former patients, and it may enable us to institute a more aggressive therapy in the latter patients, thereby achieving a higher initial rate of complete responses.

These aggressive, or salvage, treatments should use combination regimens including VP-16-213, an epipodophyllotoxin highly active in resistant germ cell tumors. Combined with ADM and DDP, this VP-16-213-based regimen provided a second complete remission in 1 of our patients who had relapsed. Used extensively by the University of Indiana Group with a good rate of remissions (Williams, *this volume*), this combination may be considered as second-line chemotherapy for patients relapsing on PVB. Perhaps, with the introduction of more active regimens, VP-16-213 could be included in combinations indicated as first-line therapy in high-risk patients.

It is important to consider the incidence of responses obtained in advanced seminomas. Even though this tumor has a greater sensitivity to radiotherapy, chemotherapy with PVB is as active and should be used in high-risk cases (with or without radiotherapy).

The single, most important prognostic factor is the extent of disease at initiation of therapy. This observation was confirmed in our patients: the incidence of complete remission was less in advanced cases and none of the patients with minimum disease suffered relapse.

Based on our results we would like to present some conclusions about the therapeutic management of advanced germ cell tumors:

1. PVB is an effective combination chemotherapy regimen for advanced germ cell tumors. Given at full doses, this combination can obtain a high complete response rate.

2. Patients not achieving complete response after three to four cycles of PVB must be considered resistant and treated with other chemotherapy.

3. Patients in partial remission with resectable residual tumor after PVB must be treated with surgery.

4. Extragonadal germ cell tumors are less responsive than gonadal tumors, with a complete response rate of 46% in our hands.

5. Patients with nonseminomas and seminomas have the same complete remission rate with PVB. This chemotherapy must be considered for primary treatment in high-risk primary seminomas patients.

6. The second-line chemotherapy regimen with VP-16 is very active in relapsing or nonresponding patients and should be considered for inclusion in first-line therapy in further studies.

REFERENCES

1. Ansfield, F. J., Korbitz, B. D., Davis, H. L., Jr., and Ramirez, G. (1969): Triple therapy in testicular tumors. *Cancer*, 24:442–446.
2. Bosl, G. J., Kwong, R., Lange, P. H., Fraley, E. E., and Kennedy, B. J. (1980): Vinblastine intermittent, bleomycin, and single-dose cis-dichlorodiammineplatinum (II) in the management of Stage III testicular cancer. *Cancer Treat. Rep.*, 64:331–334.
3. Einhorn, L. H. (1980a): Chemotherapy of metastatic seminomas. In: *Testicular Tumors, Management and Treatment*, edited by L. H. Einhorn, p. 151. Masson Publishers USA, New York.
4. Einhorn, L. H. (1980b): Extragonadal germ cell tumors. In: *Testicular Tumors, Management and Treatment*, edited by L. H. Einhorn, Masson Publishers USA, New York.
5. Einhorn, L. H., and Donohue, J. (1977): Cis-diamminedichloroplatinum, vinblastine, and bleomycin combination chemotherapy in disseminated testicular cancer. *Ann. Int. Med.*, 87:293–298.

6. Einhorn, L. H., and Williams, S. D. (1980): Chemotherapy of disseminated testicular cancer. *Cancer*, 46:1,339–1,344.

7. Feun, L. G., Samson, M. K., and Stephens, R. L. (1980): Vinblastine (VLB), bleomycin (BLEO), cis-diamminedichloroplatinum (DDP) in disseminated extragonadal germ cell tumors. *Cancer*, 45:2,543–2,549.

8. Golbey, R. B., Reynolds, R. F., and Vugrin, D. (1979): Chemotherapy of metastatic germ cell tumor. *Semin. Oncol.*, 6:82–87.

9. Higby, D. J., Wallace, H. J., Albert, D. J., and Holland, J. F. (1974): Diamminedichloroplatinum: A phase I study showing responses in testicular and other tumors. *Cancer*, 33:1,219–1,225.

10. Hong, W. K., Wittes, R. E., Hajdu, S. T., Cvitkovic, E., Whitmore, W. F., and Golbey, R. B. (1977): The evolution of mature teratoma from malignant testicular tumors. *Cancer*, 40:2,987–2,992.

11. Johnson, D. E., Bracken, R. B., Ayala, A. G., and Samuels, M. L. (1978): Retroperitoneal lymphadenectomy as adjunctive therapy in selected cases of advanced testicular carcinomas. *J. Urol.*, 116:66–68.

12. Kennedy, B. J. (1970): Mithramycin therapy in advanced testicular neoplasm. *Cancer*, 26:755–766.

13. Li, M. C., Whitmore, W. F., Golbey, R., and Grabstald, H. (1960): Effects of combined drug therapy on metastatic cancer of the testis. *JAMA*, 174:145–153.

14. MacKay, E. N., and Sellers, A. H. (1966): A statistical review of malignant testicular tumors based on the experience of the Ontario Cancer Foundation Clinics, 1938–1961. *Can. Med. Assoc. J.*, 94:889–899.

15. MacKenzie, A. R. (1966): Chemotherapy of metastatic testis cancer results in 154 patients. *Cancer*, 19:1,369–1,376.

16. Mañas, A., Cubillo, S., Alonso, A., Moyano, A., Cabello, A., and Cortes Funes, H. (1979): Monitoring peripheral neurotoxicity from cis-platinum (DDP). In: *Medical Oncology*, Springer International (Abstract), 124:31.

17. Merrin, C., Takita, H., Weber, R., Wajsman, A., Baumgartner, G., and Murphey, G. P. (1976): Combination radical surgery and multiple sequential chemotherapy for the treatment of advanced carcinoma of the testis (Stage III). *Cancer*, 37:20–29.

18. Mostofi, F. K. (1973): Proceedings: Testicular tumors, epidemologic, etiologic, and pathologic features. *Cancer*, 32:1,186.

19. Moyano, A., Mañas, A., Ramos, A., Mendiola, C., Usera, G., and Cortes Funes, H. (1979): Renal toxicity to different cumulative doses of cis-platinum (DDP). In: *Medical Oncology*. Springer International (Abstract), 140:35.

20. Peckham, M. J., Barret, A., McElwain, W. F., and Raghavan, D. (1981): Nonseminoma germ cell tumors (malignant teratoma) of the testis: Results of treatment and analysis of prognostic factors. *Br. J. Urol. (in press)*.

21. Samson, M. K., Fisher, R., Stephens, Rivkin, S., Opipari, M., Maloney, T., and Groppe, C. W. (1980): Vinblastine, bleomycin, and cis-diamminedichloroplatinum in disseminated testicular cancer: Response to treatment and prognostic correlation. A Southwest Oncology Group Study. *Eur. J. Cancer*, 16:1,359–1,366.

22. Samuels, M. L., and Howe, C. D. (1970): Vinblastine in the management of testicular cancer. *Cancer*, 25:1,009–1,017.

23. Samuels, M. L., Johnson, E. E., and Holoye, P. U. (1975): Continuous intravenous bleomycin therapy with vinblastine in stage III testicular neoplasia. *Cancer Chemother. Rep.*, 59:563–570.

24. Samuels, M. L., Lanzotti, V. J., Holoye, P. Y., and Howe, C. D. (1977): Stage III testicular cancer: Complete response by substage to velban plus continuous bleomycin infusion (VB-3). *Proc. Am. Assoc. Cancer Res.*, 18:146.

25. Stoter, G., Sleijfer, D., Vendrik, C. P. I., Schraffort Koops, H., Struyrenberga, A., Van Oosterom, A. T., Brouwers, T. H. M., and Pinedo, H. M. (1979): Combination chemotherapy with cis-diamminedichloroplatinum, vinblastine, and bleomycin in advanced testicular nonseminoma. *Lancet*, 1:941–945.

26. Willis, G. W., and Hajdu, S. I. (1973): Histologically benign teratoid metastasis of testicular embryonal carcinoma: Report of five cases. *Am. J. Clin. Pathol.*, 59:388–393.

27. Wyatt, J. K., and McAninch, L. H. (1967): A chemotherapeutic approach to advanced testicular carcinoma. *Cancer J. Surg.*, 10:421–426.

New Approaches in Cancer Therapy,
edited by H. Cortés Funes and M. Rozencweig.
Raven Press, New York © 1982.

VP-16 Salvage Therapy for Refractory Germ Cell Tumors: An Update

Stephen D. Williams and Lawrence H. Einhorn

Department of Medicine, Indiana University Medical Center and the Indianapolis Veteran's Administration Medical Center, Indianapolis, Indiana 46223

The dramatic advances made in the management of testis germ cell tumors in the last decade are well known. Quite realistically, virtually all patients with early stage disease (7) and about 60 to 70% of patients with disseminated disease (2) can be cured by modern therapy. However, there remains a significant proportion of patients with metastatic disease who fail to be cured. Thus, investigations of secondary treatment regimens are appropriate.

Prior to 1978 at Indiana University, patients who failed to attain complete remission with four courses of platinum + vinblastine + bleomycin ± adriamycin (PVB ± A) or those who relapsed from complete remission were treated with a variety of secondary platinum-containing regimens. Although most attained a further objective response, there were no cures. At the same time, we saw a small group of patients who had failed prior vinblastine + bleomycin treatments. They were treated with platinum + adriamycin (3). Objective responses were frequent, but no patients experienced long, disease-free survival.

At about this time, the single agent activity of VP-16-213 in germ cell tumors was recognized. Current single-agent data for this drug are shown in Table 1. In our experience, this is the only drug ever to induce objective response in patients refractory to platinum. Accordingly, we incorporated this drug in combination regimens for pretreated patients with testis and extragonadal germ cell tumors. This chapter will update our previously published experience (8) with these patients.

TABLE 1. *VP-16 in testicular cancer*

Institution	Response/total	Ref.
EORTC	6/30	1
Royal Marsden/Charing Cross	11/24	5
Indiana/Vanderbilt	3/5	7 and S. D. Williams (unpublished data)
Total	20/59 (33.9%)	

PATIENTS AND METHODS

From 1978 to 1980, 45 previously treated patients were treated with platinum + VP-16 combination regimens. The various regimens used are shown in Table 2. The regimen used for an individual patient was based on his prior chemotherapy history. For example, the regimen of choice was the four-drug program, but patients who had previously exhibited progressive disease on one or more of these agents did not receive this drug; likewise, if the patient had previously received 450 mg/m² of adriamycin or had findings of bleomycin lung disease, these agents were not used.

After completion of induction therapy, if residual disease was present, it was surgically resected, if feasible. Subsequently, for these patients and those in complete remission, three monthly maintenance courses were given and then therapy was terminated. Patients were followed every 1 or 2 months with chest X-ray and marker determinations. Remission duration and survival are dated from initiation of chemotherapy.

The characteristics of the patient population are shown in Table 3. As can be seen, they tended to be heavily pretreated, and 42 had received prior platinum. Many patients had received multiple prior treatment regimens.

Table 4 shows the extent of disease in these patients according to the criteria of Samuels (6). As expected, the majority (73.3%) had advanced disease.

Complete remission was defined as the disappearance of all radiographically documented disease and normalization of markers. Partial remission was defined as a 50% decrease in measurable disease or, if none was present, a return of significantly elevated marker levels to normal.

RESULTS

Table 5 shows the distribution of the treatment regimens given. As there were no obvious differences between the results obtained from the different regimens, they will be considered as a group.

As expected, the toxicity in this heavily treated patient population was substantial. Twelve patients (27.9%) required hospitalization for fever and granulocytopenia,

TABLE 2. *Treatment regimens*[a]

DDP, 20 mg/m² daily for 5 days
+
VP-16, 100 mg/m² i.v. daily for 5 days
±
Adriamycin, 40 mg/m² i.v. push day 1
±
Bleomycin, 30 units i.v. push weekly
Maintenance: VP-16, 300 mg/m² i.v. q 4 weeks

[a]Courses given every 3 weeks for three–four courses with continuous saline hydration.

TABLE 3. *Patient population*

	No. of patients
Cell type	
Embryonal	21
Teratocarcinoma	17
Chorio	2
Seminoma	5
	45
Prior therapy[a]	
Radiation	14
DDP combinations	
1	35
2	7
Vlb + bleo	6
Other	10

[a]Many patients had multiple prior treatments.

TABLE 4. *Extent of disease*

A: Minimal pulmonary	6	
B: Advanced pulmonary	17	
C: Minimal abd. ± pulmonary	2	33 (73.3%)
D: Advanced abdominal	16	
E: Elevated marker only	1	
Other	3	
Total	45	

TABLE 5. *Distribution of treatment regimens*

DDP + VP-16	4
DDP + VP-16 + Bleo	13
DDP + Adr + VP-16 + Bleo	23
DDP + Adr + VP-16	5
Total	45

with 6 having clinical or microbiologic evidence of infection. Seven patients (16.3%) had severe thrombocytopenia (<25,000). Eleven patients (25.6%) had clinical or radiographic evidence of bleomycin-induced pulmonary disease. The drug was discontinued promptly in these patients and in no case was of lasting significance. There was 1 drug-related death in a patient with prior radiation who developed severe myelosuppression after his first course and died of sepsis and bleeding.

Response to therapy, remission duration and survival, and current status are shown in Table 6. Overall, 24 patients attained disease-free status, with 17 (37.8%) continuously free of disease and 18 presently NED. All have been followed for a

TABLE 6. *Response, duration, survival*

Response	Number (%)	Relapse
Complete remission	11 (24.4)	1
Partial remission	30 (66.7%)	
NED with surgery	13 (28.9%)	
Teratoma[a]	7	1
Carcinoma[a]	6	5
None	1 (2.2%)	
Early death[b]	3 (6.7%)	
Continuously NED	17 (37.8%)	
Presently NED	18 (40.0%)	
Range 15–42 months (median = 32.5)		
Median follow-up (range) = 32.5 months		
(15–42 months)		
Followed 1 + year	18	
Followed 2 + year	14	

[a]Pathologic findings of postchemotherapy resection.
[b]One drug death; 2 due to disease.
NED, no evidence of disease.

minimum of 1 year and 14 for at least 2 years. Of note, 5/6 patients who were rendered disease-free by resection of residual carcinoma relapsed and died, usually very soon after surgery and frequently before postoperative chemotherapy could be initiated.

Although the numbers are small, it appeared that minimal disease and a history of a prior complete remission increased the likelihood of having a durable complete remission with salvage therapy. Also, the length of time since that last course of platinum prior to salvage therapy appeared directly related to the likelihood of complete remission.

No patient has relapsed later than 1 year after initiation of salvage therapy.

DISCUSSION

Additional follow-ups and patients reaffirm our initial report of the effectiveness of platinum + VP-16 for refractory germ cell tumors. It is now clear that about ⅓ of such patients will be cured by this approach which, we believe, is a most striking and gratifying therapeutic response.

Toxicity was considerable, but acceptable in view of the results. However, one possibility for reduction of hematologic toxicity and mucositis would be the omission of adriamycin. We believe this may be done for the following reasons: (a) Although the numbers are small in this study, there was no obvious difference in the various regimens; (b) Our most recent study (4) in new patients had not shown any value for PVB + A versus PVB; and (c) Prior to 1978, platinum ± adriamycin ± vincristine and bleomycin was used for pretreated patients. There were no long survivors.

Thus, we believe that platinum + VP-16 ± bleomycin is an established regimen for refractory patients. It is the therapy of choice for the type of patients treated in this study and, since there are, to our knowledge, no long disease-free survivors in such patients without VP-16, the use of this agent is mandatory. In addition, we plan to investigate the use of this regimen in new patients in a random prospective trial as compared to platinum + vinblastine + bleomycin.

VP-16 is an active drug in germinal neoplasms and represents a significant therapeutic advance for certain types of patients.

ACKNOWLEDGMENTS

Supported in part by Southeastern Cancer Study Group Grant #CA-19657 and PHS MO1 RR00 750-06.

REFERENCES

1. Cavalli, F., Klepp, O., Renard, J., Röhrt, M., and Alberto, P. (1981): A phase II study of oral VP-16-213 in nonseminomatous testicular cancer. *Eur. J. Cancer*, 17:245–249.
2. Einhorn, L. H., and Donohue, J. P. (1979): Combination chemotherapy in disseminated testicular cancer: The Indiana University experience. *Semin. Oncol.*, 6:87–93.
3. Einhorn, L. H., and Williams, S. D. (1978): Combination chemotherapy with cis-dichlorodiam-mineplatinum (II) and adriamycin for testicular cancer refractory to vinblastine plus bleomycin. *Cancer Treat. Rep.*, 62:1351–1353.
4. Einhorn, L. H., Williams, S. D., Turner, S. (1981): The role of maintenance therapy in disseminated testicular cancer: A Southeastern Cancer Study Group protocol. *Proc. Am. Soc. Clin. Oncol. (Abstract)*, 22:463.
5. Fitzharris, B. M., Kaye, S. B., Saverymuttus, S., Newlands, E. S., Barrett, A., Peckham, M. J., and McElwain, T. J. (1980): VP-16-213 as a single agent in advanced testicular tumors. *Eur. J. Cancer*, 16:1,193–1,197.
6. Samuels, M. L., Lanzotti, V. S., Holoye, P., Boyle, P. Y., Smith, T. L., and Johnson, D. E. (1976): *Cancer Treat. Rev.*, 3:185–204.
7. Williams, S. D., Einhorn, L. H., and Donohue, J. P. (1980): High cure rate of stage I or II testicular cancer with or without adjuvant therapy. *Proc. Am. Soc. Clin. Oncol. (Abstract)*, 21:421
8. Williams, S. D., Einhorn, L. H., Greco, F. A., Oldham, R., and Fletcher, R. (1980): VP-16-213 salvage therapy for refractory germinal neoplasms. *Cancer*, 46:2,154–2,158.

New Approaches in Cancer Therapy,
edited by H. Cortés Funes and M. Rozencweig.
Raven Press, New York © 1982.

Hormonochemotherapy Versus Hormonotherapy Followed by Chemotherapy in the Treatment of Disseminated Breast Cancer

*F. Cavalli, **P. Alberto, †F. Jungi, ‡K. Brunner, and §G. Martz

*Division of Oncology, Ospedale San Giovanni, Bellinzona; **Division of Oncology, Hôpital Cantonal, Genève; †Division of Oncology, Kantonsspital, St. Gallen; ‡Division of Oncology, Inselspital, Bern; and §Division of Oncology, Kantonsspital, Zürich, Switzerland

Chemotherapy and hormonal therapy act by different mechanisms and have different spectra of toxicity. It would seem promising to combine both modalities in the treatment of advanced breast cancer with the hope of improving results, since combination chemotherapy seems to have reached a plateau in effectiveness (5,6).

In a previous study of the Swiss Group for Clinical Cancer Research (SAKK), the combined modality approach with simultaneous polychemotherapy and hormonal treatment did not produce statistically significant better results than did chemotherapy alone (3). However, there was a clear-cut tendency for better remission, longer remission duration, and survival when chemotherapy was combined with oophorectomy in premenopausal patients.

The study detailed in this chapter has therefore been directed toward the question: Should combination chemotherapy be delayed until primary failure under hormonal therapy or should both treatments be started simultaneously? The second option relates to the correlation between "aggressiveness" of the chemotherapy and therapeutic results. In fact, there have been suggestions (8) that even a low-dose chemotherapy can achieve results similar to those produced by more toxic combinations. Moreover, as already mentioned, chemotherapy for breast cancer seems to have reached a plateau in effectiveness. We therefore designed our study to be able to answer the following question also: How aggressive should the first combination chemotherapy used in previously untreated patients with metastatic breast cancer be?

MATERIAL AND METHODS

The protocol (SAKK 2/75) was activated within the participating institutions (Division of Clinical Oncology of the Cantonal and University Hospital of Geneva, Lausanne, Bern, Basel, Zürich, St. Gallen, and Bellinzona) late in 1975. The study design is outlined in Table 1. Before random assignment to treatment groups, patients were classified according to menopausal status and to "risk group" ["low" or "high" risk, based on a retrospective evaluation of previous SAKK studies (2)]. The following cases were considered to be "low risk":

1. Free interval (FI) mastectomy-diagnosis of the first metastasis of at least 2 years and only contralateral, locoregional nodal metastases.
2. FI at least 2 years and only bony metastases.
3. Maximally two out of the following parameters:
   a. Lung or liver metastases (not both!) with an FI of at least 4 years.
   b. An isolated bony metastasis with an FI of at least 2 years.
   c. Scattered skin metastases (not cancer en cuirasse!) and/or an ipsilateral malignant pleural effusion of at least 2 years.
   d. Ipsilateral locoregional nodal metastases and FI of at least 2 years.

All other patients were considered "high risk."

Patients were assigned randomly to the A group (concurrent chemo- and hormonotherapy) or to the B group (hormonotherapy, observation of 6 to 8 weeks, then chemotherapy unless hormonotherapy had already produced tumor regression. If so, combination chemotherapy was started only upon new progression of the tumor parameters).

At the time of random assignment to A or B treatment groups, patients were also randomly allocated to three different chemotherapy regimens: I, II, and III. Dosage and schedule of the three regimens are shown in Table 2. Regimen I (LMFP, "minimal") is a peroral, intermittent combination designed in a pilot study carried out in St. Gallen (11). In all regimens we used chlorambucil (CLB) instead of cytoxan, in order to avoid some of the toxicities related to the latter. In a previous study the SAKK has shown that both drugs are equivalent in the treatment of breast cancer (4). Regimen II (LMP/FVP, "medium") corresponds to the "Swiss version"

TABLE 1. *Study design using the SAKK 2/75 protocol. Groups A and B are subdivided into pre/postmenopausal and low-/high-risk patients*

Group A [hormonotherapy plus chemotherapy]
    I: LMFP
    II: LMP/FVP
    III: LMFP/ADM

Group B [hormonotherapy; observation for 6–8 weeks; chemotherapy (unless remission)]
    I: LMFP
    II: LMP/FVP
    III: LMFP/ADM

Hormonotherapy: (1) Premenopausal: oophorectomy; (2) Postmenopausal: tamoxifen 10 mg BID.
See Table 2 for abbreviations.

TABLE 2. *Chemotherapy regimens*

I: Minimal (LMFP) CLB 5 mg/m²/d d 1–14 p.o. MTX 10 mg/m²/w d 1 + 8 p.o. (1 dose!) 5-FU 500 mg/m²/w d 1 + 8 p.o. PDN 30 mg/m²/d d 1–14 then ↓	q 4 weeks, intermittent
II: Medium (LMP/FVP) CLB as in I MTX 15 mg/m²/w Subdivided in 3 daily doses d 1–3, d 8–10 p.o. PDN 30 mg/m²/d d 1–14 5-FU 500 mg/m²/w d 15 + 22 i.v. VCR 1.2 mg/m²/w d 15 + 22 i.v. PDN 30 mg/m²/d d 25–28 then ↓	q 4 weeks, continuous
III: Maximal (LMFP/ADM) CLB as in I MTX 40 mg/m²/w d 1 + 8 i.v. 5-FU 600 mg/m²/w d 1 + 8 i.v. PDN 30 mg/m²/d d 1–14, then ↓ ADM 60 mg/m² d 28	q 8 weeks, intermittent

Abbreviations: ADM, adriamycin; CLB, chlorambucil; 5-FU, 5-fluorouracil; MTX, methotrexate; PDN, prednisone; VCR, vincristine.

(3,4) of the "Cooper regimen." Regimen III (LMFP/ADM, "maximal") is an alternating combination with adriamycin (ADM) and LMFP (= CMFP, but with CLB instead of cytoxan).

At the last evaluation (Feb. 15, 1980), 416 patients were entered into the study. All had measurable, previously untreated, advanced breast cancer. At this cut-off, 356 cases were already evaluable (>6 weeks of treatment), 20 were too early for evaluation, and 41 were not evaluable (protocol violations, refusal of patients, early death, etc.). Only death within 4 weeks was considered early death; deaths after 4 weeks were counted as failures.

The distribution of the pretreatment patient characteristics is shown in Table 3. Only evaluable cases are accounted for. We analyzed age, FI, menopausal status (96 pre-, 260 postmenopausal), risk group of seven sites of predominant metastases (locoregional, skeletal, locoregional + pleural effusion, locoregional + skeletal, visceral + locoregional, visceral + skeletal, and visceral only). As can be seen from Table 3, there is a very similar distribution of all characteristics between A and B groups and also among the regimens I, II, and III.

Criteria of response were the same as those used internationally: partial response (PR), no change (NC), and progressive disease (PD), except that we still use the category minor response (MR), in order to compare the current results with our previous studies. MR is defined as a clear-cut tumor shrinkage, which does not reach the limit of 50% in the sum of the product of the two largest diameters of all measurable lesions.

TABLE 3. *Pretreatment patient characteristics*

	Group		Regimen		
	A	B	I	II	III
Median age (yr)	57	59	59	58	57
Median FI (MT)	26.5	26	29	22	23.5
<12 MT[a]	27	36	26	39	31
12–60 MT[a]	56	47	60	45	49
>60 MT[a]	17	17	14	16	20
Premenopausal (N = 96)	26	25	28	26	27
Postmenopausal[a] (N = 260)	74	75	72	74	73
High risk[a]	23	26	26	25	23
Low risk[a]	77	74	74	75	77
Site of metastases[a]					
Locoregional	7	13	11	9	9
Skeletal	18	18	18	17	22
Locoregional + pleural	4	4	3	5	5
Locoregional + skeletal	18	20	12	21	21
Visceral + locoregional	12	7	14	6	10
Visceral + skeletal	27	25	24	31	20
Visceral	14	13	18	11	13

[a]Percentage.

Performance status (0 to 4) and toxicity (0 to 2) were recorded according to ECOG scale. The same grading was used in order to reduce the dosage in presence of myelosuppression (toxicity 1 = reduction 50%: toxicity 2 = reduction 100%).

Rather than duration of remission, whose onset can always conceal a subjective error, we analyze responding patients (PR, MR, and NC) according to the time from the beginning of the treatment until appearance of new progression (time-to-progression). Survival and time-to-progression were calculated based on the method of Kaplan and Meier (10).

RESULTS

Of the 356 evaluable patients, 177 were randomized in A (concurrent hormono- and chemotherapy) and 179 in B ("delayed" chemotherapy). In this latter group, 45 patients underwent an oophorectomy and 129 postmenopausal patients received tamoxifen. The therapeutic responses to oophorectomy were as follows: 7 PR (15%) and 8 MR (18%). Tamoxifen elicited 22 PR (18%) and 15 MR (11%). Both treatments are known to produce in unselected patients a remission in about ¼ of the cases. This percentage is reached in our study, if we add PR and MR. The rather low rate of PR is probably due to the stringent criteria of our protocol.

The median time to progression for patients responding to hormonotherapy only (PR + MR) was 16.0 months after oophorectomy and 17.0 months after tamoxifen.

Table 4 presents the remission rates for groups A and B. For the latter group, the results achieved with the "delayed" chemotherapy are added to the tumor regressions produced by the hormonotherapy; but patients who achieved a second chemotherapy-induced remission after a first hormonotherapy-induced regression are accounted for only once.

Concerning the actuarial survival, in the premenopausal group there is a statistically not-significant difference ($p = 0.09$) in favour of A (27.2 months median survival versus 21.5 for B), whereas in the postmenopausal group, an essentially similar difference ($p = 0.22$) is found for B (32.2 months) versus A (23.5 months).

In Table 5 are summarized the remission rates according to the chemotherapy regimens (I = LMFP, II = LMP/FVP, III = LMFP/ADM) for the 318 patients who are already evaluable as regards this treatment modality. These 318 cases encompass essentially all evaluable patients of the concurrent hormonochemotherapy group (A), whereas for the B group ("delayed" chemotherapy) we recorded all chemotherapy-treated cases, either after primary or secondary failure to hormonotherapy. As it can be seen, the "maximal" regimen (III) and "medium" regimen (II) together are superior ($p < 0.05$) to the "minimal" chemotherapy (I). A detailed report of the side effects of the three different chemotherapy regimens is not possible here. We note, however, that haematologic and nonhaematologic toxicities are both significantly ($p < 0.05$) more pronounced concerning frequency and intensity in regimen III when compared to those of the LMFP-chemotherapy. The combination LMP/FVP shows an intermediate score of toxicity.

Concerning the actuarial survival according to the three different chemotherapy regimens, the median survival times in months are: 28.1 for I, 24.2 for II, and 28.5 for III. These results are essentially similar ($p = 0.8$).

DISCUSSION

We present here an interim evaluation of a still ongoing trial. We are continuing the study because we hope that, by accruing more patients, we will be able to substantiate some differences in different subsets of patients.

For the time being, we can only partially confirm two previous reports, in which premenopausal patients fared significantly better when combination chemotherapy was immediately added to oophorectomy (1,9). In our study, in fact, the differences as regards remission rate, time-to-progression, and survival are in favour of the group with concurrent oophorectomy-chemotherapy. But the disadvantage for the

TABLE 4. *Therapeutic results*

Group	No. of patients	Partial response[a]	Minor response[a]
Premenopausal			
A	51	27 (53%)	7 (14%)
B	47	17 (36%)	17 (36%)
Postmenopausal			
A	126	53 (42%)	16 (13%)
B	132	45 (34%)	28 (21%)

[a]See text for response criteria.

TABLE 5. *Therapeutic results: chemotherapy*

| | | Response rate (%) | |
| | | Partial | Minor |
Regimen	No. of patients	response[a]	response[a]
I	107	24	19
II	103	46	15
III	108	44	18
Total	318		

I vs. (II + III): $p = 0.001$.
[a]See text for response criteria.

premenopausal patients with "delayed" chemotherapy lacks statistical significance. It must be emphasized, however, that in at least one of the two mentioned reports (1), statistically significant differences were found only after exclusion of the group with early progression. The other report has so far been presented only as an abstract without elaborate statistical analysis (9).

We want also to stress a methodological difference between our trial and the above mentioned studies. In our study the "delayed" chemotherapy was begun, unless tumor regression was apparent 6 to 8 weeks after oophorectomy or start of tamoxifen, in postmenopausal women. The two other studies called for the beginning of "delayed" chemotherapy only in case of evident tumor progression after oophorectomy.

We are not aware of a similar study in postmenopausal patients. Contrary to the first evaluation of our trial (7), at present we have essentially the same remission rate for patients treated simultaneously with tamoxifen and chemotherapy and for cases with "delayed" chemotherapy. However, as regards survival, there seems to be an advantage emerging in favour of the group with "delayed" chemotherapy. The difference so far lacks statistical significance, but is becoming more evident in each subsequent analysis of our trial.

The second question investigated in our study relates to the problem of dose-response relationship in the treatment of advanced breast cancer (12). The interpretation of our present results is difficult. In fact, we have clear differences with more and better tumor regressions in favour of the more aggressive and toxic regimens. In the overall study population, we have also a stringent relationship between the grade of the therapeutic response and the median survival. But the survival curves so far are similar for all three chemotherapy regimens. A possible answer to this intriguing question could be that there are different therapeutic responses to the subsequent treatments among relapsing patients. It is, in fact, possible that the great majority of patients relapsing after a "maximal" chemotherapy (in our study, LMFP/ADM) are resistant to a secondary treatment. On the other hand, we have some evidence in favour of the hypothesis that at least a significant subset of the patients receiving a "minimal" chemotherapy (in our study, LMFP) is still responsive to a later, more intensive combination chemotherapy. But to answer this question properly, we must await a final and thorough evaluation of our study.

REFERENCES

1. Ahmann, D. L., O'Conell, M. J., Hahn, R. G., Bisel, H. F., Lee, R. A., and Edmonson, J. H. (1977): An evaluation of early or delayed adjuvant chemotherapy in premenopausal patients with advanced breast cancer undergoing oophorectomy. *N. Engl. J. Med.*, 297:356.
2. Brunner, K. W. (1978): Stand der Hormon-und Chemotherapie beim Mammakarzinom. *Schweiz. Med. Wschr.*, 108:1,338.
3. Brunner, K. W., Sonntag, R. W., Alberto, P., Senn, H. J., Martz, G., Obrecht, P., and Maurice, P. (1977): Combined chemo- and hormonal therapy in advanced breast cancer. *Cancer*, 39:2,923.
4. Brunner, K. W., Sonntag, R. W., Martz, G., Senn, H. J., Obrecht, P., and Alberto, P. (1975): A controlled study in the use of combined drug therapy for metastatic breast cancer. *Cancer*, 36:1,208.
5. Carbone, P. P., Bauer, M., Band, P., and Tormey, D. (1977): Chemotherapy of disseminated breast cancer. Current status and prospects. *Cancer*, 39:2,916.
6. Carbone, P. P., and Davis, T. E. (1978): Medical treatment for advanced breast cancer. *Semin. Oncol.*, 4:417.
7. Cavalli, F., Alberto, P., Jungi, F., Martz, G., and Brunner, K. W. (1978): Tamoxifene alone or combined with multiple drug chemotherapy in disseminated breast cancer. *Current Chemotherapy, Tenth International Congress on Chemotherapy*, p. 1,286. American Society of Microbiology, Washington, D.C.
8. Creech, R. H., Catalano, R. B., Mastrangelo, M. J., and Engstrom, P. F. (1975): An effective low-dose intermittent cyclophosphamide, methotrexate, and 5-fluorouracil treatment regimen for metastatic breast cancer. *Cancer*, 35:1,101.
9. Falkson, G., Falkson, H. C., Leone, L., Glidwell, O., Weinberg, V., and Holland, J. F. (1978): Improved remission rates and durations in premenopausal women with metastatic breast cancer. A Cancer and Acute Leukemia Group B study. *Proc. ASCO*, 19:416.
10. Kaplan, E. L., and Meier, P. (1958): Nonparametric estimation from incomplete observations. *J. Am. Stat. Ass.*, 53:457.
11. Senn, H. J., Fopp, M., and Amgwerd, R. (1979): Divergent effect of adjuvant chemoimmuno-therapy on recurrence rates in node-negative and -positive breast cancer patients. *Proc. ASCO*, 20:393.
12. Tattersall, M. H., and Tobias, J. S. (1977): Are dose-response relationships relevant in clinical cancer chemotherapy? *In Recent Advances in Cancer Treatment*, edited by H. J. Tagnon and M. J. Staquet, p. 227. Raven Press, New York.

New Approaches in Cancer Therapy,
edited by H. Cortés Funes and M. Rozencweig.
Raven Press. New York © 1982.

Breast Cancer Studies at the Milan Cancer Institute: The Combined Modality Experience

P. Valagussa, A. Rossi, G. Tancini, C. Brambilla, S. Marchini, and G. Bonadonna

Istituto Nazionale Tumori, Milano, Italy

Despite the evolution of therapeutic research, the management of cancer of the breast still represents one of the most serious challenges in oncology. Innumerable disputes continue about the optimal treatment strategy, since breast cancer is indeed a complex mosaic of diseases, even at its early stages. In fact, the classic approach based on anatomical principles [radical mastectomy (RM) ± postoperative irradiation] has reached a plateau in the cure rate of primary breast cancer.

A full knowledge of the natural history of the disease remains, therefore, the only possible way towards a better understanding of the magnitude of the problem. Findings reported by the NSABP group (11) and the Milan Institute (18) have provided insight into important questions. The histologic status of axillary lymph nodes proved to be the single most reliable prognostic factor: the 10-year relapse-free survival (RFS) of women with positive axillary nodes ($N+$) was in the range of 25% as compared to 75% for patients with negative nodes. Although the RFS was not affected by menopausal status, it was inversely proportional to the size of primary tumor, especially in patients with $N+$ (18). Furthermore, the likelihood of developing distant metastases within a short period after surgery in the majority of $N+$ patients (18) provided ample explanation for the inability of local-regional modalities to control the disease effectively. This finding, in fact, strongly supported the assumption that distant micrometastases were already present prior to diagnosis.

By the late 1950s, laboratory research had shown that clinically available drugs used in some mammalian species prevented or delayed recurrences after operation (13). More recently, similar experiments have demonstrated that a higher cure rate was possible when treatment was delivered shortly after surgery (16).

Based on the above reported findings, a new generation of prospectively randomized clinical trials were started at the beginning of the 1970s. In September 1972, under the chairmanship of B. Fisher, the NSABP launched a study aimed at evaluating the efficacy of a single drug chemotherapy [L-phenylalanine mustard (L-PAM)] in preventing recurrences in women operated on for primary breast cancer and with $N+$ (10). In the same direction, a study was activated in June 1973 at

109

the Milan Institute using a three-drug combination known as CMF (cyclophosphamide, methotrexate, and fluorouracil) (2).

It is important to emphasize that these were the first two studies with the appropriate design to test the validity of an adjuvant treatment in patients with $N+$. In
fact, only patients in whom a complete clearance of the axillary nodes was performed
at the time of RM and in whom there was histologic evidence of cancer invasion
were eligible for entry into the study. After surgery, women were stratified according
to age and number of involved nodes and were randomly allocated to receive either
no further treatment or adjuvant chemotherapy: L-PAM for 18 courses in the NSABP
protocol; CMF for 12 monthly cycles in the Milan trial. Furthermore, base-line
studies should have excluded the presence of distant metastases, and no other
antineoplastic treatment (e.g., postoperative radiotherapy and/or hormone manip-
ulations) could be administered. With this trial design, should a benefit have become
evident, it no doubt was due to the treatment under investigation and not to other
variables (e.g., different stages of disease, other concomitant treatments, etc.).

The aim of this chapter is to summarize the results achieved so far in the first
CMF program and in the subsequent combined modality studies carried out at the
Milan Institute.

FIRST CMF PROGRAM

As already mentioned, the first CMF study was started in June 1973 with the
aim to evaluate the efficacy of an adjuvant triple combination in increasing both
the relapse-free survival (RFS) and overall survival compared to RM alone.

Study design, patient characteristics, treatment plan, follow-up studies, and timing, as well as short and intermediate analyses, have been systematically published
during the past few years (2,3,7,15). Table 1 summarizes the results achieved at
5 years from radical mastectomy. Adjuvant CMF was able to alter the course of

TABLE 1. *First CMF program: 5-year results*

	RM (179)		CMF (207)		
	%	Median duration (mos)	%	Median duration (mos)	p
RFS: Total	44.6	35	59.5	NR[b]	0.0005
1–3 nodes	48.1	44	69.4	NR	<0.0005
>3 nodes	33.0	16	40.5	42	<0.06
Premenopause	43.4	30	65.9	NR	<0.0005
Postmenopause	49.3	45	55.7	NR	0.22
Overall survival	66.2	NR	78.4	NR	0.04
Second malignancies					
Contralateral breast ca.	2.2		2.9		
Other neoplasms[a]	1.7		0.9		

[a]No. patients with leukemia.
[b]NR: Median not reached.

operable breast cancer compared to patients treated only with RM. The 5-year RFS was 59.5% compared to 44.6% ($p = 0.0005$). This was especially true for patients with one to three nodes and for premenopausal women. In the subgroup with more than three nodes, even if there was not a clear statistically significant difference ($p < 0.06$), there was a strong evidence of a beneficial effect of adjuvant chemotherapy, since the median RFS of the CMF-treated patients was more than double that of the control group (42 months versus 16 months). Apparently, there was no advantage for CMF-treated postmenopausal women.

There was also evidence of an improved overall survival in women given adjuvant chemotherapy ($p = 0.04$). The 5-year analysis indicated that second-line treatment at first relapse yielded comparable results between patients initially treated with RM and RM + CMF (15), suggesting that in relapsing breast cancer, salvage therapy seems to be ineffective.

CMF: 12 VERSUS 6 CYCLES

The intent of the second CMF program (17) was to test whether six cycles of CMF could yield results similar to those obtained with a longer treatment duration. In fact, at that time, there was no information regarding the optimal duration of an adjuvant treatment. Between September 1975 and May 1978, a total of 459 patients were entered into the study and randomized to receive either 12 or 6 cycles of CMF. Accrual for postmenopausal women was discontinued in March 1977 because the 3-year analysis of the previous study had indicated that CMF was apparently ineffective in this subgroup (3). All other criteria for eligibility and stratification parameters remained unchanged.

Findings from the 4-year analysis are now available and have indicated that, in patients given 12 cycles, the results between the first and second study were almost superimposable. Therefore, all women randomized to receive 12 cycles were grouped together (total: 450 patients) and data are reported in Table 2, comparing the groups treated with CMF and the control group of the previous study. The essential findings can be summarized as follows: (a) There were no significant differences in both

TABLE 2. *CMF 12 vs 6: 4-year results[a]*

	RM (179)	CMF 12[b] (450)	CMF 6 (216)
RFS: Total	48.4	62.7	69.4
1–3 nodes	53.2	76.8	77.5
>3 nodes	36.5	43.6	56.9
Premenopause	44.2	66.5	69.4
Postmenopause	52.4	57.4	68.8
Overall survival	75.2	79.4	82.1

[a]Data are in percents.
[b]First study: RFS 62.5, overall survival 81.9.
Second study: RFS 62.7, overall survival 76.8.

the RFS and overall survival rates between the groups given 12 or 6 cycles. However, there was a trend in the RFS in favor of patients given 6 cycles compared to those treated with 12 cycles for women with > three nodes and in the postmenopausal category ($p = 0.13$ and $p = 0.22$, respectively). (b) The RFS of patients given either 12 or 6 cycles was superior to the RFS of patients treated only with RM. The difference was statistically significant for the total series of patients and for the subgroups with one to three nodes and in the premenopausal category. Also, the RFS of women with > three nodes and given 6 cycles of CMF was statistically superior to the results achieved in the control group, whereas, in the remaining subsets, there was only a trend in favor of CMF-treated patients.

SEQUENTIAL COMBINATIONS

With the aim of testing a more aggressive form of drug treatment in postmenopausal women, in May 1977 a new trial utilizing two non-cross-resistant regimens [CMF + prednisone (P) for six cycles followed by four cycles of adriamycin + vincristine (AV)] was initiated (7,9). In the attempt to evaluate in humans the Norton-Simon hypothesis (14), patients were randomly allocated to receive sequential combinations either with no dose intensification (i.e., full doses from the first cycle) or with progressive intensification (i.e., drugs were given at low dose during the first two cycles and were progressively escalated every two cycles). In this particular study, no dose reduction schedule was planned, but, in the presence of myelosuppression, treatment was delayed until full marrow recovery occurred. Entry into the study was limited to postmenopausal women aged 65 years or less and with no medical contraindication to an adriamycin-containing regimen. The preliminary 2-year results from a total of 115 patients are reported in Table 3. Contrary to initial observations (9), available findings indicate that there was no difference between the two types of administration (no intensification versus intensification). A preliminary comparison with results achieved in patients of the same age group and entered in our previous studies, while confirming a beneficial effect of adjuvant treatment over patients treated only with RM (2-year RFS: total group, 64.6%; one to three nodes, 69.4%; > three nodes, 54.8%), seems to indicate that there was not a clear advantage of sequential combinations as compared to CMF alone, with the exception of women with one to three nodes treated with an initial full dose (96.1% versus CMF 12: 85% versus CMF 6: 82.7%). However, it should be stressed that it is premature to make a meaningful comparison.

TABLE 3. *CMFP-AV: Percent 2-yr RFS in postmenopausal women ≤ 65 years*

	No intensification	Intensification
Total	83.0	78.6
1–3 nodes	96.1	90.8
>3 nodes	67.0	66.9

ANCILLARY STUDIES

CMF and Amenorrhea

Combination chemotherapy with CMF can induce amenorrhea in about 70% of menstruating women. This finding, coupled with the apparent discrepancy of results between pre- and postmenopausal women, contributed to the question of whether the beneficial effect obtained in CMF-treated premenopausal patients could be due to some hormonal changes. As already reported (7), the 5-year analysis of the first CMF study has also confirmed that drug-induced amenorrhea is not tantamount to chemical castration (5). In fact, in the two major age groups, the results observed in patients with and without amenorrhea were superimposable: in women ≤ 40 years, the 5-year RFS was 42.1% for patients with and 41.3% for women without amenorrhea. In patients > 40 years, the findings were 73.1% and 75%, respectively. Also, there was no difference when degree of nodal involvement and duration of amenorrhea (transient versus irreversible) were considered. All these findings further minimize the possible therapeutic role of drug-induced chemical castration (5).

Adjuvant CMF and Estrogen Receptor Status

Estrogen receptor (ER) determination on the primary tumor was carried out, at the time of surgery, in a large fraction of women who were part of the second adjuvant program (CMF 12 versus 6 cycles). The comparative analysis at 4 years essentially confirmed our previous observation (8). Findings reported in Table 4 indicate that there was no significant difference in the RFS of ER + and ER − tumors; this held true in all subgroups. On the contrary, overall survival of ER + premenopausal women was significantly superior to that of ER − patients. Even if a proper comparison with results obtained in patients not given adjuvant chemotherapy is not possible, our findings suggest that the benefit achieved with adjuvant CMF was independent from ER status and support evidence against the hypothesis that ER − tumors could be more responsive to combination chemotherapy.

Dose-Response Relationship

A recent analysis has extensively evaluated the possible role of dose level in the outcome of results in patients treated with adjuvant CMF (4). When subgroups of

TABLE 4. *4-yr percent RFS and overall survival after adjuvant CMF related to ER status*

	ER +	ER −	*p*
Premenopause			
RFS	69.8	59.4	0.18
Survival	80.3	70.9	<0.04
Postmenopause			
RFS	61.7	59.3	0.41
Survival	84.4	76.5	0.48

patients who received comparable drug dosages were analyzed separately, there was evidence that results in pre- and postmenopausal women were superimposable and that the best results were obtained in patients given $\geq$ 85% of the planned dose (level 1). On the contrary, women who received < 65% of the dose (level 3) had an RFS that was almost superimposable on that of patients treated only with RM (Table 5). Postmenopausal women given CMF received overall a lesser amount of drugs (64.1%) as compared to premenopausal women (75.9%); the overall results (total CMF, Table 5) reflect this fact. Furthermore, within each dose level, the results were related to the number of involved nodes and, within each patient subgroup with a certain number of nodes, the 5-year RFS was dose related; this held true both for pre- and postmenopausal women (Table 5). These findings suggest that, as already reported for animal model systems (16), at the clinical level there is also a dose-response relationship, at least in human breast cancer.

The above reported results were derived from patients randomized to receive 12 cycles of CMF either in the first or in the second study. A similar dose-response relationship was evident in patients who received 6 cycles of CMF (6). These data suggest that, although there will probably be a correlation between the total amount of CMF administered and the RFS, the peak levels of the drugs given is an important pharmacological factor.

Treatment Morbidity

Acute toxicity from adjuvant CMF has been reported in detail in previous publications (2,3,17). Suffice it to say that we did not observe any drug-related deaths, and severe and/or prolonged episodes of myelosuppression were not documented.

As far as chronic organ damage is concerned, an accurate evaluation of possible liver toxicity from methotrexate administration has revealed that, at the doses given in the combination, it was unable to cause any significant hepatic alteration (1). Furthermore, as clearly shown in Table 1, the 5-year analysis failed to detect an increased incidence of second neoplasms in patients given adjuvant CMF compared to patients treated only with RM.

TABLE 5. *5-yr RFS related to dose levels: 12 CMF cycles[a]*

CMF level	Premenopause			Postmenopause		
	Total	nodes		Total	nodes	
		1–3	>3		1–3	>3
I (≥85%)	79.1	86.0	64.4	75.3	83.3	59.9
II (84–65%)	55.7	68.1	32.8	55.9	67.3	37.7
III (<65%)	45.5	55.9	23.3	48.9	57.9	27.1
Total CMF	63.6	70.2	34.5	54.1	62.9	34.2
RM	43.4	48.5	26.8	49.3	50.8	40.5

[a]First and second study.

CONCLUSION

The results reported so far clearly indicate that, by utilizing a combined modality strategy, an improvement has been achieved in operable breast cancer with N+ both in terms of RFS and overall survival. Similar observations have also been reported by other investigators with different effective regimens (12). Therefore, there is little doubt that therapeutic research is moving in the direction of a "cure" for women with breast cancer.

From the sequence of studies activated at the Milan Institute, the following observations can be made: (a) There is not a different effect of adjuvant chemotherapy in pre- and postmenopausal women, provided comparable doses are given. (b) In an adjuvant situation, when effective chemotherapy is utilized, ER status does not appear to be an important prognostic variable. (c) The only important prognostic parameter remains the degree of axillary nodal involvement, since patients with > three nodes have the worst prognosis even after adjuvant treatment. (d) A short-term chemotherapy (i.e., approximately six cycles) is able to achieve control of the disease, provided the drugs used in the combination are effective and given at therapeutic doses.

To further improve the cure rate of operable breast cancer, however, an entirely new generation of clinical trials, such as those currently ongoing in Milan, should be activated. They will provide the answer to the many unsolved problems, such as: (a) optimal treatment regimen (drugs, doses, and schedule); (b) optimal treatment duration; (c) efficacy of non-cross-resistant regimens; (d) efficacy of combined chemohormonal treatments in patients with ER+; and (e) identification of subgroups that can really benefit from adjuvant treatments (all N+ patients? high-risk N− patients?).

Meanwhile, proper efforts should also be directed toward improvement of the quality of patient life by exploring the possibility of lesser surgical procedures and determining the cost-benefit ratio (including long-term morbidity, and psychosocial and economical problems) of systemic adjuvant therapy. Time is essential for solving the problem of optimal treatment strategy in breast cancer, but cooperation among different research institutions is equally important to achieve the goal.

ACKNOWLEDGMENT

This work was supported in part by Contract NO1-CM-33714 with the Division of Cancer Treatment, National Cancer Institute, NIH, Bethesda, Maryland.

REFERENCES

1. Bajetta, E., Buzzoni, R., Giardini, R., and Bonadonna, G. (1981): Liver assessment in women receiving adjuvant CMF chemotherapy. *Tumori*, 67:27–30.
2. Bonadonna, G., Brusamolino, E., Valagussa, P., Rossi, A., Brugnatelli, L., Brambilla, C., De Lena, M., Tancini, G., Bajetta, E., Musumeci, R., and Veronesi, U. (1976): Combination chemotherapy as an adjuvant treatment in operable breast cancer. *N. Engl. J. Med.*, 294:405–410.
3. Bonadonna, G., Rossi, A., Valagussa, P., Banfi, A., and Veronesi, U. (1977): The CMF program for operable breast cancer with positive axillary nodes. Updated analysis on the disease-free interval, site of relapse, and drug tolerance. *Cancer*, 39:2904–2915.

4. Bonadonna, G., and Valagussa, P. (1981): Dose-response effect of adjuvant chemotherapy in breast cancer. *N. Engl. J. Med.*, 304:10–15.
5. Bonadonna, G., Valagussa, P., and De Palo, G. (1981): The results of adjuvant chemotherapy in breast cancer are predominantly due to the hormonal change such therapy induces. The view against. In: *Controversies in Medical Oncology*, edited by M. B. Van Scoy-Mosher, pp. 100–109. G. K. Hall & Co., Boston.
6. Bonadonna, G., Valagussa, P., Rossi, A., Tancini, G., Brambilla, C., Marchini, S., and Veronesi, U. (1981): Multimodal therapy with CMF in resectable breast cancer with positive axillary nodes. The Milan Institute experience. In: *Adjuvant Therapy of Cancer, III*, edited by S. E. Jones, and S. E. Salmon, pp. 435–444. Grune & Stratton, New York.
7. Bonadonna, G., Valagussa, P., Rossi, A., Zucali, R., Tancini, G., Bajetta, E., Brambilla, C., De Lena, M., Di Fronzo, G., Banfi, A., Rilke, F., and Veronesi, U. (1978): Are surgical adjuvant trials altering the course of breast cancer? *Semin. Oncol.*, 5:450–464.
8. Bonadonna, G., Valagussa, P., Tancini, G., and Di Fronzo, G. (1980): Estrogen receptor status and response to chemotherapy in early and advanced breast cancer. *Cancer Chemother. Pharmacol.*, 4:37–41.
9. Brambilla, C., Valagussa, P., Bonadonna, G., and Veronesi, U. (1980): Sequential adjuvant chemotherapy in postmenopausal ($\leqslant$ 65 yrs) breast cancer. *Proc. Am. Assoc. Cancer Res.*, 21:189.
10. Fisher, B., Carbone, P., Economou, S. G., Frelick, R., Glass, A., Lerner, H., Redmond, C., Zelen, M., Band, P., Katrych, D. L., Wolmark, N., Fisher, E. R., and other Cooperative Investigators (1975): L-phenylalamine mustard (L-PAM) in the management of primary breast cancer. A report of early findings. *N. Engl. J. Med.*, 292:117–122.
11. Fisher, B., Slack, N., Katrych, D. L., and Wolmark, N. (1975): Ten-year follow-up results of patients with carcinoma of the breast in a cooperative trial evaluating surgical adjuvant chemotherapy. *Surg. Gynecol. Obstet.*, 140:528–534.
12. Jones, S. E., and Salmon, S. E., editors (1981): *Adjuvant Therapy of Cancer. III.* Grune & Stratton, New York.
13. Martin, D. S. (1959): An appraisal of chemotherapy as an adjuvant to surgery for cancer. *Am. J. Surg.*, 97:685–686.
14. Norton, L., and Simon, R. (1977): Tumor size, sensitivity to therapy, and design of treatment schedules. *Cancer Treat. Rep.*, 61:1307–1317.
15. Rossi, A., Bonadonna, G., Valagussa, P., and Veronesi, U. (1981): Multimodal treatment in operable breast cancer: Five-year results of the CMF programme. *Br. Med. J.*, 282:1427–1431.
16. Schabel, F. M., Jr. (1977): Rationale for adjuvant chemotherapy. *Cancer*, 39:2875–2882.
17. Tancini, G., Bajetta, E., Marchini, S., Valagussa, P., Bonadonna, G., and Veronesi, U. (1979): Preliminary 3-year results of 12 versus 6 cycles of surgical adjuvant CMF in premenopausal breast cancer. *Cancer Clin. Trials*, 2:285–292.
18. Valagussa, P., Bonadonna, G., and Veronesi, U. (1978): Patterns of relapse and survival following radical mastectomy. Analysis of 716 consecutive patients. *Cancer*, 41:1170–1178.

New Approaches in Cancer Therapy,
edited by H. Cortés Funes and M. Rozencweig.
Raven Press, New York © 1982.

Laparotomy with Therapeutic Intent After 6 Months of Induction Chemotherapy for Bulky Ovarian Cancer

*Steven E. Vogl, **Vicki Seltzer, **Antonio Canalog,
**Mamdouh Moukhtar, †Fernando Camacho, *Barry H. Kaplan,
and †Edward Greenwald

*Departments of *Medicine and **Gynecology, Albert Einstein College of Medicine,
Bronx, New York 10461; and †Department of Oncology, Montefiore Hospital and
Medical Center, Bronx, New York 10467*

The identification of cis-diamminedichloroplatinum II (DDP) as an active agent in advanced ovarian cancer led to 5 years of intense activity in the development of new treatments for this disease incorporating this active agent. Its use has led to dramatic improvements in remission rates and in the quality of the remissions achieved by chemotherapy. Wiltshaw and Kroner were the first to identify DDP as a useful drug in the treatment of ovarian cancer, producing objective responses in 26% of women whose tumors had worsened despite alkylating agent chemotherapy (12). Hexamethylmelamine (HXM), with 25%, is the only other agent that produces responses in more than 20% of patients after failure of alkylating agent chemotherapy (11). In an effort to improve these low response rates, with median response durations of only 4 months for patients refractory to alkylating agents, we combined these two agents with adriamycin (ADM), an antibiotic shown to approximate melphalan in its activity against ovarian cancer in patients without prior chemotherapy (2). A combination of these three drugs, given the acronym "HAD," produced responses in 53% of patients whose tumors were refractory to alkylating agent therapy, with a median response duration of 6 months (8). Hematologic toxicity with the combination was considerable, not because high doses were used, but because all patients had extensive prior chemotherapy, together with radiation therapy in 35%. In spite of the relatively high response rate (higher than that generally reported for melphalan as initial chemotherapy), no patient was cured by the HAD regimen given after failure of an alkylating agent. It should be noted that all patients entered had bulky tumors which were easily evaluable for response.

After the HAD trial was begun, several studies clearly demonstrated a lack of efficacy for ADM as a single agent in ovarian cancer after failure of alkylating agents (1,3,5). We then increased the dose of DDP to 75 mg/m² every 3 weeks together with 200 mg/m² of HXM given in the 2nd and 3rd week of each 3-week cycle (a regimen given the acronym "HD-75") and achieved a 55% response rate with 24% complete remissions. The median duration of remission was 8 months, and 2 of the patients who achieved complete remission remain free of disease for more than 2 years (6).

The high rate of significant and relatively long remissions achieved using HXM and DDP in patients refractory to alkylating agents led us to design a regimen combining these drugs with an alkylating agent for initial chemotherapy of advanced (stage 3 and 4) ovarian cancer. We expected the drugs to be tolerated better in this patient population, since bone marrow reserve would not be impaired by prior chemotherapy and since patients would have lesser tumor burdens and a better general state of health. It was elected to combine the HAD drugs with an alkylating agent because alkylating agents have been shown to cure some women with ovarian cancer (4), and data demonstrating curative potential for other drugs are not available. Cyclophosphamide (CTX) was chosen as the alkylating agent because it is readily administered i.v., is more sparing of megakaryocyte function than other alkylating agents, has less cumulative marrow toxicity than other alkylating agents, and is synergistic in animal tumor model systems with both ADM and DDP.

The i.v. drugs (CTX, ADM, and DDP) were given once each cycle to maximize convenience and to avoid making the patient vomit several times a month from the repeated administration of DDP. Cycles were repeated only every 4 weeks in order to allow marrow recovery and so deliver full doses repeatedly to most patients. DDP was administered at a dose of 50 mg/m^2 in a 2-hr program of hydration with 2 liters of fluid (5% dextrose in 0.45% saline with 10 mEq KCl per liter) and diuresis with furosemide and mannitol, which has been shown to prevent almost entirely clinically significant nephrotoxicity (10). HXM (150 mg/m^2) was administered orally in divided doses daily for 2 weeks beginning 8 days after the administration of the i.v. drugs. This was done so that all patients would have recovered from the nausea induced by DDP prior to beginning a potentially nauseating oral drug such as HXM. The dose of HXM was adjusted downward if nausea was produced. The schema for this program, given the acronym "CHAD," is shown in Table 1.

The initial results of the CHAD pilot study were remarkable. Of 26 patients evaluable for response, 24 (92%) clearly responded, with complete clearing of all clinical signs and symptoms of disease in 11 (42%) (9). The benefits proved transitory, however, for most of those patients who entered with bulky tumors. The

TABLE 1. *The CHAD regimen*

Drug	Dosage	Day 1	8	21
CTX	600 mg/m^2 i.v.	×		
HXM	150 mg/m^2 p.o.		× × × × × × × × × × ×	
ADM	25 mg/m^2 i.v.	×		
DDP	50 mg/m^2 i.v.	×		

median time-to-disease-progression for those who achieved partial remission was only 8 months, whereas the median time-to-disease progression for those with complete remission was 24 months. At this time, with 3 years of follow-up, only 2 of 11 complete responders are still free from relapse. The best prognosis was shared by 12 patients who began chemotherapy without sufficient bulky tumor to be evaluated for response. In this patient population, the median time-to-disease progression is in excess of 3 years.

Cox regression analysis both of time-to-disease-progression and survival revealed that the only significant prognostic factor for either endpoint was tumor bulk at the time the patient began chemotherapy. If the largest tumor diameter was 3 to 10 cm, median time-to-disease progression was 15 months, and if the largest tumor diameter was >10 cm, it was 8 months.

Survival followed a similar pattern. Median survival for patients with tumor diameters ≤2 cm at entry has not been reached. It was 22 months for those with tumor diameters 3 to 10 cm, and 11 months for patients with tumors >10 cm in diameter.

Preliminary results of an Eastern Cooperative Oncology Group (ECOG) study confirmed the importance of tumor bulk in predicting time-to-disease progression in advanced ovarian cancer (7). In this study, 253 patients were randomly assigned to receive chemotherapy either with oral melphalan or with the CHAD program. CHAD produced significantly more remissions in those patients evaluable for response (64% versus 43%, $p = 0.002$), with many more complete remissions (39% versus 19%). Among those with tumor diameters at entry greater than 10 cm, median time-to-disease progression on CHAD was 7.6 months (versus 3.4 months for melphalan). Median time-to-disease progression on CHAD was much longer, 14.3 months, if the tumor diameter was 2 to 10 cm at entry (versus 6.5 months on melphalan). The follow-up is as yet too short to comment on time-to-disease progression for patients with minimal tumor burdens at entry in the ECOG study.

The overwhelming influence of tumor bulk on the prognosis of these patients with advanced, metastatic ovarian cancer (stage 3 and 4) led us to wonder if the favorable influence of surgical resection was limited to the period just after diagnosis and before systemic therapy. We presumed that the deleterious effect of bulky tumor related to the high probability of there being resistant cells, or cells that would have resistant offspring, when large numbers of cells were exposed to initial chemotherapy. We wondered if initially unresectable masses of tumor could be resected after substantial shrinkage had been induced by chemotherapy. If this could be accomplished, perhaps relapse could be delayed or prevented by resecting sites of bulky tumor where resistant clones of tumor cells would most likely be emerging.

As shown in Figs. 1 and 2, responses to CHAD chemotherapy for most patients in the initial pilot study were prompt, but many patients required five or even six cycles of chemotherapy before they achieved their best remissions. In order to give the surgeon the best chance of resecting previously unresectable tumors, laparotomy was deferred until after the sixth cycle of chemotherapy. We recognized that only those patients with better partial remissions or complete remissions would get to

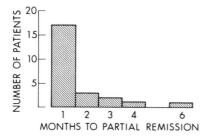

FIG. 1. Time to achieve partial remission in the 24 patients who achieved remission in the original CHAD pilot series.

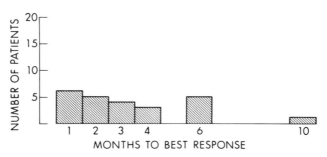

FIG. 2. Time to achieve maximal tumor regression (complete remission or best partial remission) from start of CHAD therapy for the 24 responding patients in the original CHAD pilot series.

this point. It is a fair assumption that any large tumor nodule remaining at this point would contain large populations of drug-resistant cells, so that a surgical procedure to remove such nodules is reasonable. Even major surgery could be justified, since the prognosis of such patients must be very poor.

We sought first, therefore, to determine the feasibility of late removal of bulky tumor when it had not been possible to reduce the tumor burden effectively at initial laparotomy. Second, we were interested in determining if removal of this bulky tumor led to any apparent improvement in the prognosis of the patient. Third, we wondered if completing the standard surgical procedure (total abdominal hysterectomy and bilateral salpingo-oopherectomy) in patients with some or all of the organs remaining after first surgery would be of value.

MATERIALS AND METHODS

Eligibility was restricted to women with stage 3 and 4 epithelial ovarian cancer with metastases beyond the brim of the true pelvis. All patients had to have tumor diameters >2 cm at the time of entry and had to be out of bed at least once a day. The white blood count had to be greater than 4,000/μl, the platelet count greater than 100,000/μl, the serum creatinine less than 1.5 mg/dl, and there had to be no clinically significant cardiac disease. Informed consent was obtained from each patient.

The treatment program consisted of an induction period of six cycles of CHAD chemotherapy (Table 1) given at 28-day intervals. Between 4 and 7 weeks after the start of the sixth cycle, patients were brought to the operating room and a laparotomy was performed. The abdomen was inspected and palpated. If no gross tumor was noted, multiple biopsies were obtained. If possible, any and all areas of tumor involvement were resected. If the uterus or either ovary had not been removed at an earlier procedure, removal was accomplished, if this was technically feasible.

Therapy after laparotomy was to include DDP, HXM, and CTX plus concurrent low-dose whole abdominal irradiation. Radiation was added to the chemotherapy program in an effort to inhibit replication of drug-resistant clones, prolong remission, and increase, perhaps, cure rate. Initially, 150 rads were given to the whole abdomen on 3 consecutive days followed by i.v. CTX and DDP and oral HXM beginning 1 week later. Such cycles were to be repeated five times, provided hematologic toxicity was not excessively prolonged. Later, as it became clear that the combination of radiation and chemotherapy was safe and produced no significant toxicity except that on the bone marrow, the radiation schedule was changed so that 150 rads were given in seven fractions over 9 days immediately following a dose of DDP (50 mg/m^2) and followed in 4 days by a 2-week course of HXM (150 mg/m^2 per day). If bone marrow recovery occurred by 5 or 6 weeks, a second cycle of 1,050 rads with DDP and HXM was given. After the completion of radiation therapy, further chemotherapy was administered with CTX, HXM, and DDP in the same schedule as CHAD, with the doses reduced if myelosuppression occurred. The details of this program, and its impact, will be published separately.

PATIENTS

Nineteen patients entered the trial. Two were excluded from further analysis. One of these had a primary endometrial cancer (not ovarian cancer) with extension to the cervix and parametrial tissues. At second laparotomy, after achieving partial remission, the other excluded patient was found to have a pancreatic cancer with normal ovaries. In this case, the histological findings at the initial laparotomy had not been strongly suggestive of an ovarian primary.

The median age of the remaining 17 patients was 61, with a range of 41 to 79. Four patients were under 50 and 3 were past their 70th birthday. Three were performance status 0 (fully active) at the time they began chemotherapy, 7 were ambulatory with symptoms (performance status 1), 3 were bedridden less than half the day (performance status 2), and 4 were bedridden more than half the day (performance status 3). Four had metastases outside the abdominal cavity at the time of entry, and the rest were stage 3. The tumors were papillary serous cystadenocarcinomas in 15 patients, solid adenocarcinoma in a single patient, and endometrioid carcinoma in a single patient. Tumor was well differentiated in 1 patient, poorly differentiated in 9 patients, and had intermediate differentiation on Broders' scale in 10 patients.

Initial surgery consisted of total abdominal hysterectomy and bilateral salpingo-oopherectomy plus omentectomy in only 3 patients. Five had bilateral salpingooopherectomies, together with omentectomy in 2. One had a unilateral oopherec-tomy and an omentectomy, and 7 had biopsies only as their initial procedures.

Induction chemotherapy lasted 6 months in 12 of the 17 patients. It lasted 5 months in 1, 7 months in 1, and 8 months in 3. Delays until second laparotomy were due either to difficulties in scheduling an operating room or to late marrow recovery after the last cycle of chemotherapy, or both. Three patients were not evaluable for response to initial chemotherapy because no sites of disease could be readily followed. Of the remaining 14 patients, 4 had complete clearing of all clinical evidence of disease, 9 had clear-cut partial remissions (greater than 50% decrease in the products of perpendicular diameters of measurable lesions), and 1 had apparent stable disease (at laparotomy, only microscopic residual tumor was later found in this patient, so she did, in fact, have an excellent response).

RESULTS

Two patients had no palpable, visible, or histologic evidence of tumor at second laparotomy. An additional 4 patients had only microscopic evidence of residual tumor, though necrotic or granulomatous areas were sometimes visible at laparotomy. Gross evidence of residual tumor was obvious at surgery in 11 patients.

Table 2 ranks the patients according to largest tumor diameter at the conclusion of the first laparotomy and states the procedures performed during each laparotomy and the residual tumor burden at the end of each operative exercise.

Six-month laparotomy failed to reduce the tumor burden substantially in 16 out of 17 patients. There was no gross tumor to resect in 6 patients (patients 5 and 9 had not even microscopic evidence of tumor in nine biopsies in each case, and patients 1, 7, 9, and 13 had only microscopic viable tumor). Thus, because of the efficacy of 6 months of CHAD therapy, these 6 patients could not possibly have late resection of bulky tumor, because no bulky tumor remained.

Of 11 patients with palpable tumor masses at the start of the second procedure, only 1 had resection of all gross tumor (patient 13). Two patients (4 and 14) had numerous nodules <1 cm in diameter throughout the peritoneal cavity both before and after the procedure. A single patient (patient 3) had partial resection of a pelvic mass, so that largest tumor nodule was 0.5 instead of 1.5 cm in diameter, and is doing well 6 months later. This resection represented a very small reduction in the total tumor burden of this patient. Four patients had partial excision of residual tumor masses, so that the largest remaining nodule was approximately 2 cm in diameter (patients 2, 6, 11, and 12). These patients, unfortunately, all relapsed soon after the second procedure (1, 1.5, 2, and 9 months later). This suggests that the remaining tumor was already composed largely of drug-resistant cells. Once drug resistance was established, partial resection of tumor was of no benefit.

No significant reduction of massive tumor burdens was possible in 3 patients (10, 15, and 17), 2 of whom promptly relapsed (after 3 and 4 months); follow-up remains short for the 3rd.

In summary, only 1 patient was moved by second laparotomy from the category of bulky tumor to one of low tumor burden. Reducing tumor bulk to the level of

TABLE 2. *Effect of first and second laparotomy on tumor bulk*

Patient number	Initial procedure	Second procedure	Maximum tumor diameter at:			Months from second laparotomy to:	
			End of first lap	Second lap		Disease progression	Death
				Start	Finish		
1	TAH, BSO, omentx	bx	3cm	micro	micro	19+	19+
2	BSO	exc	3	3	2	9	12
3	TAH, BSO, omentx	exc	4	1.5	0.5	6+	6+
4	BSO	omentx	5	0.4	0.4	10	11
5	BSO, omentx	TAH	5	0[a]	0	14+	14+
6	omentx	TAH, BSO	7.5	3	2	1.5	9
7	bx	TAH, BSO, omentx	8	micro	micro	5+	5+
8	TAH, BSO, omentx	bx	12	0[a]	0	4+	4+
9	BSO, omentx	TAH	>10	micro	micro	22+	22+
10	bx	omentx	>10	>10	>10	4+	4+
11	BSO, omentx	exc	>10	6	2	1	16
12	USO, omentx	exc	12	4	2	2	6
13	bx	TAH, BSO	15	5	micro	14+	14+
14	bx	TAH, BSO	15	0.8	0.3	3+	3+
15	bx	bx	15	15	15	2	2+
16	BSO	bx	20	micro	micro	3	21
17	bx	TAH, BSO, excX2	20	15	15	4	4

[a]All biopsies negative for tumor.

Abbreviations: Micro, microscopic disease only; omentx, omentectomy; exc, excision of tumor mass(es); TAH, total abdominal hysterectomy; B(or U)SO, bilateral (unilateral) salpingo-oopherectomy; lap, laparotomy.

masses 2 cm in diameter was of no apparent value in 4 patients. The 3 patients with massive tumor (>10 cm in diameter) after 6 months of CHAD all proved, once again, to have unresectable tumors. Finally, 6 patients, 3 of whom had massive tumors at the end of first laparotomy, had no gross tumor to resect after 6 months of CHAD.

Two patients with only microscopic residual tumor and 3 patients with gross residual tumor had total abdominal hysterectomy and bilateral salpingo-oopherectomy at the time of the second laparotomy. An additional 2 patients, 1 with microscopic residual tumor and 1 with no residual tumor, who had previously had both ovaries resected, now had a total abdominal hysterectomy. Even with limited follow-up, it is now clear that resecting the uterus and ovaries and leaving cancer ≥2-cm diameter is useless—both such patients relapsed after 1.5 and 4 months. Follow-up is too short for the remaining 5 patients to make any statement as to the potential value of late resection of the uterus and ovaries. We note that of 14 patients with the uterus in place after first laparotomy, only 7 had it resected at second laparotomy.

Major complications of surgery were noted after 2 of 17 second laparotomies (12%): 1 pulmonary embolism and 1 rectus sheath abscess requiring later surgical drainage. An additional patient had a minor wound infection delaying subsequent therapy by 2 weeks.

CONCLUSIONS

The effort to resect bulky tumor after maximal response to chemotherapy was a failure. It was accomplished only in 1 of 17 patients (6%). The lack of success was due both to the efficacy of chemotherapy in leaving no gross tumor (35%) or small tumor burdens (18%) and to the failure of the surgical procedure to reduce residual bulky tumor to < 2 cm in diameter (41%).

We may have chosen the wrong patients for second-effort surgical resection of bulky tumor by selecting the 6-month point. Perhaps all patients with residual bulky tumor by this point have drug resistance sufficiently widespread in the peritoneal cavity so that removing bulky tumor is either impossible or of no use. The distribution of drug resistance to small nodules could be either by metastasis from the large tumor masses or by independent induction in the smaller ones. One should remember that even a 1-cm tumor nodule harbors approximately 1,000 million cells.

We now wonder if a surgical second-effort might not be of value in a different patient population, those with massive initial tumor burdens, many of whom would relapse before 6 months of treatment have elapsed. Second-effort surgery might be useful in these patients after 2 months of CHAD, since most remaining tumor masses would be still composed largely of drug-sensitive cells. Most of the patients chosen for such a group would have had no initial resection of tumor, so that the chance of finding bulky tumor, at least in the ovaries, would be high after just 2 months of CHAD therapy.

In any case, the present study shows the almost universal futility of laparotomy with therapeutic intent after 6 months of effective chemotherapy. Longer follow-up is unnecessary to reach this conclusion, since so few patients had any significant tumor reduction at the 6-month laparotomy. Surgical resection of bulky tumor at the time of diagnosis of metastatic ovarian cancer remains the only hope for cure or even long-term remission.

ACKNOWLEDGMENTS

This work was supported in part by Public Health Service grants CA-14958, CA-13330 (National Cancer Institute), and RR-00050 (Division of Research Resources) from the National Cancer Institutes of Health, Department of Health and Social Services; by the Chemotherapy Foundation; and by the New York City Division of the American Cancer Society.

We thank Ms. Edna Owens for her invaluable assistance in data collection and retrieval and Ms. Linda Trongone for her help in preparation of the manuscript.

REFERENCES

1. Bolis, F., D'Incalci, M., Gramellini, F., and Constantino, M. (1978): Adriamycin in ovarian cancer patients resistant to cyclophosphamide. *Eur. J. Cancer*, 14:1,401.
2. DePalo, G. M., DeLena, M., DiRe, F., Luciani, L., Valagussa, P., and Bonadonna, G. (1978): Melphalan versus adriamycin in the treatment of advanced carcinoma of the ovary. *Surg. Gynecol. Obstet.*, 141:899–902.
3. Hubbard, S. M., Barkes, P., and Young, R. C. (1978): Adriamycin therapy for advanced ovarian carcinoma recurrent after chemotherapy. *Cancer Treat. Rep.*, 62:1,375.
4. Smith, J. P., Rutledge, F. N., and Delclos, L. (1975): Results of chemotherapy as an adjunct to surgery in patients with localized ovarian cancer. *Semin. Oncol.*, 2:277–281.
5. Stanhope, C. R., Smith, J. P., and Rutledge, F. (1977): Second trial drugs in ovarian cancer. *Gynecol. Oncol.*, 5:52.
6. Vogl, S. E., Pagano, M., Davis, T. E., Einhorn, N., Tunca, J., Kaplan, B. H., and Arseneau, J. C. (1981): Hexamethylmelamine and diamminedichloroplatinum in advanced ovarian cancer after failure of alkylating agent therapy. *Cancer Treat. Rep. (in press)*.
7. Vogl, S. E., Pagano, M., and Kaplan, B. H. (1981): Cyclophosphamide, hexamethylmelamine, adriamycin, and diamminedichloroplatinum "CHAD" vs. melphalan for advanced ovarian cancer— A randomized prospective trial of the Eastern Cooperative Oncology Group. *Proc. Am. Soc. Clin. Oncol.*, 22:473.
8. Vogl, S. E., Pagano, M., Kaplan, B. H., Einhorn, N., Arseneau, J., and Greenwald, E. (1980): Combination chemotherapy of advanced ovarian cancer with hexamethylmelamine, cis-platinum and adriamycin (doxorubicin) after failure of prior therapy. *Obstet. Gynecol.*, 56:635–640.
9. Vogl, S. E., Pagano, M., Kaplan, B. H., Greenwald, E., Arseneau, J., and Bennett, B. (1981): Cisplatin-based combination chemotherapy for advanced ovarian cancer: High overall response rate with curative potential only in women with small tumor burdens. *Cancer (in press)*.
10. Vogl, S. E., Zaravinos, T., Kaplan, B. H., and Wollner, D. (1981): Safe and effective two-hour outpatient regimen of hydration and diuresis for the administration of cis-diamminedichloroplatinum (II). *Eur. J. Cancer*, 17:345–350.
11. Wharton, J. T., Rutledge, F., Smith, J. P., Herson, J., and Hodge, M. P. (1979): Hexamethylmelamine: An evaluation of its role in the treatment of ovarian cancer. *Am. J. Obstet. Gynecol.*, 133:833–834.
12. Wiltshaw, E., and Kroner, T. (1976): Phase II study of cis-dichlorodiammineplatinum (II) (NSC-119875) in advanced adenocarcinoma of the ovary. *Cancer Treat. Rep.*, 60:55–60.

New Approaches in Cancer Therapy,
edited by H. Cortés Funes and M. Rozencweig.
Raven Press, New York © 1982.

Recent Trends in the Treatment of Advanced Lung Cancer

Reto Abele and Pierre Alberto

Division of Oncology, University Hospital, CH-1211 Geneva 4, Switzerland

Treatment of lung cancer is generally considered a challenge. Although activity has been observed with a large variety of antitumor agents and combinations thereof, the gloomy prognosis for most patients with advanced disease has not significantly changed over the past few years. Long-term survival for advanced disease is still exceptional. However, modern chemotherapy programs have revealed high activity, particularly in small-cell anaplastic carcinoma, and will probably improve patient survival. Recent series have pointed out prognostic factors for response to chemotherapy and survival, such as extent of disease, tumor load, performance status, and histology. Further, standardization of methods of observation and reporting should help to define more precisely the therapeutic impact of new agents or combination regimens.

Lung cancer can no longer be considered an entity. The morphologic classification modified from the World Health Organization (WHO) recognizes four main types of lung cancer (Table 1). The "oat cell" carcinoma represents the lymphocyte type of small-cell anaplastic carcinoma. Small-cell anaplastic carcinoma includes, as well, other cellular subtypes that are called intermediate. Combined types of lung cancer should be recorded separately and specified. Tumor classification helps to delineate distinct cellular biology forms that may respond differently to treatment.

TABLE 1. *Histologic classification of lung tumors*

Category	Name
10	Epidermoid carcinoma
	11. well differentiated
	12. moderately differentiated
	13. poorly differentiated
20	Small-cell anaplastic carcinoma
	21. lymphocyte-like
	22. intermediate cell
30	Adenocarcinoma
40	Large-cell carcinoma

From Matthews (41).

Small-cell carcinoma is separate from all other categories. "Non-small-cell lung cancer" is a misleading denomination that includes all the other histologic types. The characteristics and response to treatment of epidermoid, adenocarcinoma, and large-cell carcinomas are far from being identical.

Small-cell anaplastic carcinoma responds easily to many anticancer drugs. Long-term survivors (more than 2 years after diagnosis) have recently been reported. The histologic subtype of small-cell carcinoma apparently does not influence the response rate to chemotherapy (12,34). Treatment of non-small-cell tumor types remains far less successful. Responses are not frequently observed and are generally of short duration. Progress in clinical research is necessary for advanced lung cancer. This chapter will review recent series dealing with advanced stages of lung cancer. Comprehensive information may also be found in the book edited by Muggia and Rozencweig (47) and in previously published reviews (3,33).

SMALL-CELL CARCINOMA

Small-cell carcinoma is often a widely disseminated tumor at the time of diagnosis. Staging procedures determine precisely the extent of disease. Limited disease includes, by definition, tumor in one lung with possible involvement of ipsilateral hilar and supraclavicular lymph nodes; it may be treated within one radiation port. All other tumor locations are called extensive, or disseminated, disease. The extent of disease must be distinguished from tumor load, which represents the tumor bulk included in one or several sites.

A number of different drug combinations have been tested in the past few years. All these clinical trials share some common features. Combination chemotherapies with different drugs and dosages yield approximately the same global response rate in small-cell lung carcinoma. This tumor appears extremely sensitive to chemotherapy. The compounds most frequently used are cyclophosphamide, nitrosoureas, adriamycin, etoposide, and cisplatin. Combinations of three or four agents often induce higher response rates than two drugs. Further, drugs given simultaneously may give better results than sequential administration of the same drugs (5). Most trials use an intermittent schedule of administration. Antitumor agents are given over a few days, thus allowing restoration of normal tissue functions during the rest period. This type of administration allows better toxicity control by dose modification when indicated. Although intermittent schedules are most often used, a clear superiority over continuous drug administration has not been demonstrated. The majority of recent regimens use drugs at or near their maximal tolerated dose for combination chemotherapy. Increased drug dosage has also been proposed in the search for better results. The value of such an approach is still controversial and may not yield increased response rates or survivals, compared to more conventional drug dosages (1,52,63).

Chemotherapy for small-cell carcinoma has followed the usual pathways of chemotherapy development, from single-agent activity screening to combination programs. Higher response rates are progressively recorded. Complete response rates also increase, and prolongation of patient survival may be observed. Recently, a small number of patients with long-term survival has been described (36,45). At least some of these patients are candidates for cure, but a longer period of observation may be necessary (9). Good performance status, limited disease, and possibly histologic subtype (51) may favorably influence the duration of remission.

Relationship between time of entry in complete remission and duration of response or survival is largely unknown (18). The value of maintenance therapy is debated. Many authors agree that the period of treatment should not exceed 18 to 24 months, since recurrences are rare after this interval.

Table 2 shows some alternating combination regimens. Cohen et al. (18), using a high dose of lomustine (CCNU), methotrexate, and cyclophosphamide, have shown that the initial response rate may be increased by the addition of another non-cross-resistant combination of adriamycin, vincristine, and procarbazine. Complete response rate has increased in limited disease from 42 to 74%, but to a lesser degree in extensive disease. Sierocki et al. (59) have not been able to improve their results obtained with two-drug combination of cisplatin and VP-16-213 by the addition of cyclophosphamide, adriamycin, and vincristine. The value of alternating or nonalternating regimens has been randomly compared (2,4,22). No differences have been found for induction courses with cyclophosphamide, adriamycin, and etoposide, alternating or following relapses, with a CCNU, methotrexate, vincristine, and procarbazine program (2). Alternation of cyclophosphamide, CCNU, and vincristine with methotrexate, adriamycin, and etoposide in extensive disease does not improve the response rate but increases duration (22). A statistically significant survival improvement has been shown for patients treated simultaneously with a complex seven-drug combination, compared to sequential administration of the same agents given at slightly different dosages (4). Nevertheless, the impact of these therapeutic strategies on survival remains to be defined more precisely.

TABLE 2. *Alternating combination regimens for small-cell lung carcinoma*

Regimen[a] (ref.)	No. of evaluable patients[b]	Response rate (%)	
		Complete	Overall
CPA + ADM + CCNU + PRO followed by VCR + MTX + HU (4)	65	17	62
CPA + MTX + CCNU followed by VCR + ADM + PRO (18)	61	30	87
		48	93
CPA + ADM + VP-16-213 followed by CCNU + MTX + VCR + PRO (2)	45	42	82
DDP + VP-16-213 followed by CPA + ADM + VCR (59)	38	47	95
CPA + CCNU + VCR + MTX followed by ADM + VP-16-213 (22)	na	na	90[c]

[a]ADM: adriamycin; CPA: cyclophosphamide; DDP: cisplatin; HU: hydroxyurea; MTX: methotrexate; PRO: procarbazine; VCR: vincristine; VP-16-213: etoposide.
[b]na: not available.
[c]Extensive disease only.

Some simultaneous combination regimens are shown in Table 3. Hansen et al. (34) have reported that the addition of vincristine to the three-drug combination of cyclophosphamide, methotrexate, and CCNU does not improve the global response rate in advanced disease, but significantly increases the response duration (186 versus 112 days) and median patient survival (230 versus 176 days). The length of induction period may influence the remission rate, with a statistically significant difference in partial remission rates for patients receiving either two or three to six induction cycles of cyclophosphamide, adriamycin, vincristine, and etoposide (44). However, complete remission duration and survival are not dependent on the number of induction cycles. On the contrary, death rate related to treatment side effects increases with the number of induction cycles. Toxicity and morbidity induced by treatment with intensive combinations are often severe (52).

Combined Modality Treatment for Small-Cell Lung Cancer

The place of radiation therapy in the treatment of small-cell lung cancer has not been precisely determined. It should help to complete the response obtained by chemotherapy alone in limited, especially in bulky, disease. Radiotherapy may further prevent local chest recurrences. Most recent trials use radiation therapy after a chemotherapy induction (Table 4).

In a nonrandomized trial, Natale et al. (50) report a high complete remission rate in limited disease. Despite the use of radiotherapy, however, most patients have relapses within the chest after complete, unmaintained remission.

A diminution of chest recurrence incidence in patients randomly treated with or without combined modality has been shown by two groups. Overall survival has not been modified by combined treatment (22,27). In a randomized study including a small number of patients, complete remission rate is higher and relapse or death rate lower after combined treatment. No statistically significant improvement in survival has been observed (19). Radiation therapy followed by a low-dose chem-

TABLE 3. *Simultaneous combination regimens for small-cell lung carcinoma*

Regimen (ref.)	No. of evaluable patients	Response rate (%) Complete	Response rate (%) Overall
CPA + ADM + VCR (27)	84	33	80
CPA + MTX + CCNU + VCR (34)	50	na	78
CPA + MTX + CCNU (34)	48	na	75
CPA + ADM + VP-16-213 + VCR (44)	47	21	87
CPA + ADM + VP-16-213 (2)	45	40	78
CPA + ADM + VP-16-213 + VCR + DDP (50)	44	66	95
CPA + PRO + MTX + VCR (4)	30	33	73
CPA + ADM + MTX + CCNU + VCR + PRO + HU (4)	30	23	60
CPA + MTX + CCNU + VCR (22)	na	na	81[a]

[a]See Table 2 for abbreviations.

TABLE 4. *Combined modality treatment for small-cell lung carcinoma (limited disease)*

Study design (ref.)	No. of evaluable patients	Response rate (%)	
		Complete	Overall
Nonrandomized studies			
CPA ± MTX ± VCR followed by RT[a] (42)	115	40	57
CPA + VCR simultaneously with RT (62)	58	45	86
CPA + ADM + VCR + DDP + VP-16-213 followed by RT (50)	24	83	83
Randomized studies			
RT ⎰ (37)	23	30	74
RT + CPA + ADR + DTIC ⎱	24	50	75
CPA + MTX + CCNU ⎰ + RT (19)	14	77	77
⎱ − RT	14	46	46
CPA + VCR + MTX + CCNU ⎰ + RT (22)	na	na	93
⎱ − RT			85

[a]RT: radiotherapy. See Table 2 for other abbreviations.

otherapy regimen with cyclophosphamide, adriamycin, and dacarbazine (DTIC) has improved median disease-free survival in patients receiving combined treatment (27 weeks), compared to patients treated with radiotherapy alone (9 weeks) (37).

All these trials of combined modality treatment vary largely in the timing of the combination of radiotherapy with chemotherapy as well as in the dose and fractionation of radiotherapy. It is thus very difficult to draw any valid conclusions about their respective value.

Treatment toxicity induced by combined modality treatment is not negligible. When radiation and chemotherapy are not used simultaneously, reported myelosuppression seems to be tolerable. Nonhematological toxicity, in particular, early diffuse interstitial lung fibrosis, is, however, often observed (19,50). When chemotherapy is administered at the same time as radiation therapy, hematological toxicity is frequently encountered (62). Despite a maintenance treatment with chemotherapy, patients in this trial relapsed often, mostly in the chest.

Thus, response rate to combined modality treatment for limited disease is not clearly higher than to chemotherapy alone. Radiation therapy does not influence patient survival, but may prevent local recurrences.

Prophylactic brain radiation is being widely used with the intent of reducing the incidence of central nervous system involvement. However, its value for long-term disease control is debated (35,42,46). Patient overall survival is not modified by this approach.

In disseminated small-cell carcinoma, the role of radiation therapy is more difficult to determine. Thirteen responses, including 10 complete, have been obtained in 21 patients treated with a three-drug combination of cyclophosphamide, adriamycin, and vincristine with various radiotherapy programs, mostly simultaneously. Chest recurrences have been frequently seen after complete remission; all relapses were located at the site of initial bulk disease. General toxicity of this combined modality approach has been prominent (8).

"NON-SMALL-CELL" LUNG CANCER

"Non-small-cell" lung cancer includes a variety of different tumors (Table 1). Antitumor activity reported for the various histologic types is globally less pronounced than for small-cell anaplastic carcinoma. Fortunately, recent series often break down response rates according to histology. As adenocarcinoma and squamous cell carcinoma are relatively frequent compared to other types, reported activity refers, when not specified, to these two categories. Large-cell carcinoma-type is a ill-defined entity, only rarely encountered. Response to treatment in this disease is not precisely known.

Some recently published results are shown in Tables 5, 6, and 7. Most of these trials use a wide variety of different drugs in combination. Although single-drug activity has not always been studied with modern criteria, combination therapy has been used extensively in non-small-cell lung cancer. The most active two-drug

TABLE 5. *Two-drug combination therapy for non-small-cell lung carcinoma*

Regimen[a] (ref.)	No. of evaluable patients	No. of responding patients	Overall response rate (%)
DDP + DVA (14,54)	67	28	42
DDP + HMM (38)	51	8	16
DDP + VP-16-213 (6,30)	39	17	44
HMM + MMC (53)	24	4	17
DAG + ADM (23)	22	6	27

[a]DAG: dianhydrogalactitol; DVA: vindesine; HMM: hexamethylmelamine; MMC: mitomycin C.

TABLE 6. *Three-drug combination therapy for non-small-cell lung carcinoma*

Regimen[a] (ref.)	No. of evaluable patients	No. of responding patients	Overall response rate (%)
Combination with DDP			
CPA + ADM + DDP (26)	120	33	28
'' (31)	46	13	28
'' (25)	42	20	48
MMC + VLB + DDP (40)	30	16	53
DAG + ADM + DDP (23)	19	10	53
Combinations without DDP			
FU + VCR + MMC (43)	56	22	40
FU + ADM + MMC (11)	25	9	36
FU + VCR + MMC (49)	24	7	29
CPA + ADM + DVA (60)	19	5	26
CPA + ADM + VP-16-213 (66)	14	3	19

[a]FU: 5-fluorouracil; VLB: vinblastine. See Table 5 for other abbreviations.

TABLE 7. *Four- or more drug combination for non-small-cell lung carcinoma*

Regimen[a] (ref.)	No. of evaluable patients	No. of responding patients	Overall response rate (%)
Combinations with DDP			
DDP + ADM + CPA + CCNU + VCR (61)	35	23	66
DDP + MTX + BLM + ADM (65)	26	12	46
DDP + ADM + CPA + CCNU + VCR (67)	18	3	17
DDP + ADM + CPA + DVA (60)	17	6	35
DDP + MTX + BLM + VCR (56)	15	11	73
Combinations without DDP			
MTX + ADM + CPA + CCNU (17)	68	30	44
'' (64)	43	5	12
'' (20)	32	7	22
'' + VCR (39)	25	7	28

[a]BLM: bleomycin. See Tables 5 and 6 for other abbreviations.

regimens appear to be combinations of cisplatin with etoposide or vindesine. Cisplatin is synergic with several other drugs in animal systems (58). Cisplatin and etoposide form a highly active combination, especially in patients previously untreated with chemotherapy (6,30). Cisplatin in combination with vindesine also appears very promising. A 44% response rate is reported from the Memorial Sloan-Kettering Cancer Center (MSKCC) (14). Response rate does not differ for adenocarcinoma and for squamous cell carcinoma.

Other two-drug combinations appear to be of limited activity in this disease. The Mayo Clinic randomized trial showed dianhydrogalactitol and adriamycin to be statistically less active than the same agents combined with cisplatin in untreated squamous cell carcinoma. Further, a statistically significant longer duration of response and a prolonged survival have been observed with the three-drug compared to the two-drug combination (23). At the Mayo Clinic, a low dose of cisplatin (60 mg/m^2), adriamycin (40 mg/m^2), and cyclophosphamide (400 mg/m^2) given every 4 weeks has given an overall response rate of 48% in untreated patients with adenocarcinoma and large-cell carcinoma (25). The same combination but with a higher dose of cisplatin and cyclophosphamide has given a 38% response rate in squamous cell carcinoma and 27% response rate in adenocarcinoma. Responding patients had a median survival of 16 months (31). Much experience was accumulated in Canada with a CAP regimen identical to that of the Mayo Clinic. Reported response rate was only 28% for all histologies (26). It should be noted that previously treated patients were also included in this trial, which may explain the lower response rate.

Other combinations appear in Table 6. Overall response rate to three-drug combinations does not appear to be superior to those obtained with the best two-drug combinations. Drug combinations without cisplatin are also effective and may have the advantage of a better patient tolerance. Combinations of four or more drugs have been tested in relatively small series of patients (Table 7). Results vary widely but are not superior to those obtained with two-drug combinations. This fact may be related to the necessity of reducing drug dosage when simultaneously using a large number of agents. Preliminary results published by Takita et al. (61) showing a 66% overall response rate including 4 complete responses among 35 patients could not be confirmed in a smaller series testing the same combination (67). A combination of methotrexate followed by cisplatin has been reported to be very active in non-small-cell lung carcinoma without inducing significant renal toxicity (56,65).

New active drugs are needed in the treatment of non-small-cell lung cancer. Although cisplatin has been often included in combination therapy, this agent appears to play a minor role when used as single agent (7,10,15). The new vinca alcaloid vindesine appears moderately active in squamous and in adenocarcinoma histology (28,29,32,54). Chlorozotocin, a new nitrosourea analog, has been tested in various doses and schedules (13,21) and is devoid of activity in non-small-cell lung cancer. The new acridine derivate *m*-AMSA has been extensively tested at several institutions, but no significant activity has been detected for this compound, even in previously untreated patients (16,48,55,57).

CONCLUSION

Advanced lung cancer must be separated into several types from a therapeutic point of view. Small-cell anaplastic carcinoma is a rapidly progressive tumor, often widely disseminated, which responds very rapidly to many different combination therapies. Complete responses are seen frequently and prolonged patient survival has been observed. Five to 10% of treated patients are long-term survivors. Some patients may benefit from chest radiation therapy after intensive induction with chemotherapy for local disease control.

In advanced "non-small-cell" lung cancer, chemotherapy is far less active. Prolonged patient survival is only rarely observed. New agents and better and more tolerable combinations of established agents should be further tested, particularly in untreated patients. Treatment decision must weigh potential benefit for survival against known drug toxicity. Chemotherapy should be administered to only selected patients with measurable or evaluable lesions (24) and progressive disease. Protocol design must be carefully established for inclusion of a statistically sufficient patient number. Treatment of advanced lung cancer still remains an important field for clinical research.

ACKNOWLEDGMENT

The authors acknowledge the secretarial help of Ms. C. Amez-Droz.

REFERENCES

1. Abeloff, M. D., Ettinger, D. S., Khouri, N. F., and Lenhard, R. E., Jr. (1979): Intensive induction therapy for small-cell carcinoma of the lung. *Cancer Treat. Rep.*, 63:519–524.
2. Aisner, J., Whitacre, M., Van Echo, D. A., and Wiernick, P. H. (1980): Treatment of small-cell carcinoma of the lung with alternating combination chemotherapies or sequential combinations.

Abstracts, II, World Conference on Lung Cancer, edited by H. H. Hansen and P. Dombernowsky, p. 139. Excerpta Medica, Amsterdam.

3. Alberto, P. (1979): Chemotherapy as palliative treatment of primary lung cancer. *Cancer Clin. Trials*, 2:157–163.

4. Alberto, P., Berchtold, W., Sonntag, R., Barrelet, L., Jungi, F., Martz, G., and Obrecht, P. (1981): Chemotherapy of small-cell carcinoma of the lung: Comparison of a cyclic alternative combination with simultaneous combinations of four and seven agents. *Clin. Oncol.*, 17:1027–1033.

5. Alberto, P., Brunner, K. W., Martz, G., Obrecht, J. P., and Sonntag, R. W. (1976): Treatment of bronchogenic carcinoma with simultaneous or sequential combination chemotherapy, including methotrexate, cyclophosphamide, procarbazine, and vincristine. *Cancer*, 38:2,208–2,216.

6. Belgian EORTC Lung Cancer Working Party (1980): Combination chemotherapy with cisplatin (CDDP) and VP-16 in non-small-cell (NSC) bronchogenic carcinoma. *Abstracts, II, World Conference on Lung Cancer*, edited by H. H. Hansen and P. Dombernowsky, p. 116. Excerpta Medica, Amsterdam.

7. Berenzweig, M., Vogl, S. E., Kaplan, B. H., and Lanham, R. (1980): Phase II trial of cis-diamminedichloroplatinum (cDDP) in patients with non-small-cell bronchogenic carcinoma (NSCBC) not exposed to prior chemotherapy. *Proc. Am. Assoc. Cancer Res. and ASCO*, 21:457.

8. Brereton, H. D., Kent, C. H., and Johnson, R. E. (1979): Chemotherapy and radiation therapy for small-cell carcinoma of the lung: A remedy for past therapeutic failure. In: *Lung Cancer: Progress in Therapeutic Research*, edited by F. Muggia and M. Rozencweig, pp. 575–586. Raven Press, New York.

9. Brigham, B. A., Bunn, P. A., Jr., Minna, J. D., Cohen, M. H., Ihde, D. C., and Shackney, S. E. (1978): Growth rates of small-cell bronchogenic carcinomas. *Cancer*, 42:2,880–2,886.

10. Britell, J. C., Eagan, R. T., Ingle, J. N., Creagan, E. T., Rubin, J., and Frytak, S. (1978): Cis-dichlorodiammineplatinum (II) alone followed by adriamycin plus cyclophosphamide at progression versus cis-dichlorodiammineplatinum (II), adriamycin, and cyclophosphamide in combination for adenocarcinoma of the lung. *Cancer Treat. Rep.*, 62:1,207–1,210.

11. Butler, T. P., MacDonald, J. S., Smith, F. P., Smith, L. F., Woolley, P. V., and Schein, P. S. (1979): 5-Fluorouracil, adriamycin, and mitomycin-C (FAM) chemotherapy for adenocarcinoma of the lung. *Cancer*, 43:1,183–1,188.

12. Carney, D. N., Matthews, M. J., Ihde, D. C., Bunn, P. A., Jr., Cohen, M. H., Makuch, R. W., Gazdar, A. F., and Minna, J. D. (1980): Influence of histologic subtype of small-cell carcinoma of the lung on clinical presentation, response to therapy, and survival. *J. Natl. Cancer Inst.*, 65:1,225–1,230.

13. Casper, E. S., and Gralla, R. J. (1979): Phase II evaluation of chlorozotocin in patients with non-small-cell carcinoma of the lung. *Cancer Treat. Rep.*, 63:549–550.

14. Casper, E. S., Gralla, R. J., and Golbey, R. B. (1979): Vindesine (DVA) and cis-dichlorodiammineplatinum II (DDP) combination chemotherapy in non-small-cell lung cancer (NSCLC). *Proc. Am. Assoc. Cancer Res. and ASCO*, 20:337.

15. Casper, E. S., Gralla, R. J., Kelsen, D. P., Cvitkovic, E., and Golbey, R. B. (1979): Phase II study of high-dose cis-dichlorodiammineplatinum (II) in the treatment of non-small-cell lung cancer. *Cancer Treat. Rep.*, 63:2,107–2,109.

16. Casper, E. S., Gralla, R. J., Kelsen, D. P., Natale, R. B., Sordillo, P., and Houghton, A. (1980): Phase II evaluation of 4'-(9-acridinylamino)-methanesulfon-*m*-anisidine (AMSA) in patients with non-small-cell lung cancer. *Cancer Treat. Rep.*, 64:345–347.

17. Chahinian, A. P., Mandel, E. M., Holland, J. F., Jaffrey, I. S., and Teirstein, A. S. (1979): MACC (methotrexate, adriamycin, cyclophosphamide, and CCNU) in advanced lung cancer. *Cancer*, 43:1,590–1,597.

18. Cohen, M. H., Ihde, D. C., Bunn, P. A., Jr., Fossieck, B. E., Jr., Matthews, M. J., Shackney, S. E., Johnston-Early, A., Makuch, R., and Minna, J. D. (1979): Cyclic alternating combination chemotherapy for small-cell bronchogenic carcinoma. *Cancer Treat. Rep.*, 63:163–170.

19. Cohen, M. H., Lichter, A. S., Bunn, P. A., Glatstein, E. J., Ihde, D. C., Fossieck, B. E., Matthews, M. J., and Minna, J. D. (1980): Chemotherapy-radiation therapy (CT-RT) versus chemotherapy (CT) in limited small-cell lung cancer (SCLC). *Abstracts, II, World Conference on Lung Cancer*, edited by H. H. Hansen and P. Dombernowsky, p. 146. Excerpta Medica, Amsterdam.

20. Corkery, J., Wilkinson, J., Zipoli, T., Greene, R., and Lokich, J. (1980): Effective chemotherapy in non-oat cell cancer of the lung. *Proc. Am. Assoc. Cancer Res. and ASCO*, 21:449.

21. Creagan, E. T., Eagan, R. T., Fleming, T. R., Frytak, S., Kvols, L. K., and Ingle, J. N. (1979): Phase II evaluation of chlorozotocin in advanced bronchogenic carcinoma. *Cancer Treat. Rep.*, 63:2,105–2,106.

22. Dombernowsky, P., Hansen, H. H., Hansen, M., Sörensen, S., Østerlind, K., Rørth, M., and Hansen, H. S. (1980): Treatment of small-cell anaplastic bronchogenic carcinoma. Results from 2 randomized trials. *Abstracts, II, World Conference on Lung Cancer*, edited by H. H. Hansen and P. Dombernowsky, p. 149. Excerpta Medica, Amsterdam.
23. Eagan, R. T., Fleming, T. R., Frytak, S., Creagan, E. T., Ingle, J. N., and Kvols, L. K. (1980): A role of cis-dichlorodiammineplatinum (II) in squamous cell lung cancer. *Cancer Treat. Rep.*, 64:87–91.
24. Eagan, R. T., Fleming, T. R., and Schoonover, V. (1979): Evaluation of response criteria in advanced lung cancer. *Cancer*, 44:1,125–1,128.
25. Eagan, R. T., Frytak, S., Creagan, E. T., Ingle, J. N., Kvols, L. K., and Coles, D. T. (1979): Phase II study of cyclophosphamide, adriamycin, and cis-dichlorodiammineplatinum (II) by infusion in patients with adenocarcinoma and large-cell carcinoma of the lung. *Cancer Treat. Rep.*, 63:1,589–1,591.
26. Evans, W. K., Feld, R., Deboer, G., Osoba, D., Curtis, J., Pritchard, K. I., Myers, R., and Quirt, I. C. (1980): Cyclophosphamide, adriamycin, and cis-platinum in the treatment of non-small-cell lung cancer (NSCLC). *Proc. Am. Assoc. Cancer Res. and ASCO*, 21:447.
27. Fox, R. M., Tattersall, M. H. N., and Woods, R. L. (1981): Radiation therapy as an adjuvant in small-cell lung cancer treated by combination chemotherapy: A randomized study. *Proc. Am. Assoc. Cancer Res. and ASCO*, 22:502.
28. Furnas, B., Einhorn, L. H., and Rohn, R. J. (1980): A phase II trial of vindesine (DVA) in non-small-cell lung cancer (NSCLC). *Proc. Am. Assoc. Cancer Res. and ASCO*, 21:448.
29. Goldhirsch, A., Beer, M., Sonntag, R. W., Tschopp, L., Cavalli, F., Ryssel, H. J., and Brunner, K. W. (1980): Phase-II-Studie mit vindesine (desacetyl-vinblastin-amid-sulfat) bei fortgeschrittenen malignen Erkrankungen. *Schweiz. Med. Wschr.*, 110:1,063–1,067.
30. Goldhirsch, A., Joss, R., Alberto, P., Cavalli, F., and Brunner, K. W. (1980): Cis-platinum (DDP) and VP-16-213 (VP) combination with and without adriamycin (ADM) in the treatment of lung cancer. *Proc. Am. Assoc. Cancer Res. and ASCO*, 21:449.
31. Gralla, R. J., Cvitkovic, E., and Golbey, R. B. (1979): Cis-dichlorodiammineplatinum (II) in non-small-cell carcinoma of the lung. *Cancer Treat. Rep.*, 63:1,585–1,588.
32. Gralla, R. J., Raphael, B. G., Golbey, R. B., and Young, C. W. (1979): Phase II evaluation of vindesine in patients with non-small-cell carcinoma of the lung. *Cancer Treat. Rep.*, 63:1,343–1,346.
33. Greco, F. A., Einhorn, L. H., Richardson, R. L., and Oldham, R. K. (1978): Small-cell lung cancer: Progress and perspectives. *Semin. Oncol.*, 5:323–335.
34. Hansen, H. H., Dombernowsky, P., Hansen, M., and Hirsch, F. (1978): Chemotherapy of advanced small-cell anaplastic carcinoma: Superiority of a four-drug combination to a three-drug combination. *Ann. Intern. Med.*, 87:177–181.
35. Hansen, H. H., Dombernowsky, P., Hirsch, F. R., Hansen, M., and Rygard, J. (1980): Prophylactic irradiation in bronchogenic small cell anaplastic carcinoma: A comparative trial of localized versus extensive radiotherapy including prophylactic brain irradiation in patients receiving combination chemotherapy. *Cancer*, 46:279–284.
36. Hansen, M., Hansen, H. H., and Dombernowsky, P. (1980): Long-term survival in small-cell carcinoma of the lung (scc). *Abstracts, II, World Conference on Lung Cancer*, edited by H. H. Hansen and P. Dombernowsky, p. 151. Excerpta Medica, Amsterdam.
37. Krauss, S., and Perez, C. (1980): Treatment of localized undifferentiated small-cell lung carcinoma (SCLC) with radiation therapy (RT) with or without combination chemotherapy (CT) with cyclophosphamide (C), adriamycin (ADR), and dimethyltriazenoimidazole carboximide (DTIC). *Abstracts, II, World Conference on Lung Cancer*, edited by H. H. Hansen and P. Dombernowsky, p. 157. Excerpta Medica, Amsterdam.
38. Krauss, S., Tornyos, K., DeSimone, P., Lowenbraun, S., McKeown, J., Solomon, A., and Sonoda, T. (1979): Cis-dichlorodiammineplatinum (II) and hexamethylmelamine in the treatment of non-oat cell lung cancer: A pilot study of the Southeastern Cancer Study Group. *Cancer Treat. Rep.*, 63:391–393.
39. Lyman, G. H., Colledge, P., Johnson, D., and Williams, C. C. (1980): Chemotherapy of advanced bronchogenic carcinoma with methotrexate, adriamycin, cyclophosphamide, CCNU (MACC), and vincristine. *Proc. Am. Assoc. Cancer Res. and ASCO*, 21:460.
40. Mason, B. A., and Catalano, R. B. (1980): Mitomycin (M), vinblastine (V), and cisplatin (P) combination chemotherapy in non-small-cell lung cancer (NSCLC). *Proc. Am. Assoc. Cancer Res. and ASCO*, 21:447.

41. Matthews, M. J. (1973): Panel report: Morphologic classification of bronchogenic carcinoma. *Cancer Chemother. Rep.*, 4:299–301.

42. Maurer, L. H., Tulloh, M., Weiss, R. B., Blom, J., Leone, L., Glidewell, O., and Pajak, T. F. (1980): A randomized combined modality trial in small-cell carcinoma of the lung: Comparison of combination chemotherapy-radiation therapy versus cyclophosphamide-radiation therapy effects of maintenance chemotherapy and prophylactic whole brain irradiation. *Cancer*, 45:30–39.

43. Miller, T. P., McMahon, L. J., Livingston, R. B., and Moon, T. E. (1980): Extensive adenocarcinoma and large-cell undifferentiated carcinoma of the lung treated with 5-fluorouracil, vincristine, and mitomycin C (FOMi). *Proc. Am. Assoc. Cancer Res. and ASCO*, 21:453.

44. Minna, J. D., Ihde, D., Bunn, P. A., Cohen, M., Fossieck, B., and Matthews, M. J. (1980): Extensive stage small-cell carcinoma of the lung: Effect of increasing intensity of induction chemotherapy. *Abstracts, II, World Conference on Lung Cancer*, edited by H. H. Hansen and P. Dombernowsky, p. 160. Excerpta Medica, Amsterdam.

45. Minna, J., Lichter, A., Brereton, H., Bunn, P., Cohen, M., Fossieck, B., Ihde, D., Matthews, M., and Glatstein, E. (1980): Small-cell lung cancer: Long-term, potentially cured survivors in National Cancer Institute trials. *Abstracts, II, World Conference on Lung Cancer*, edited by H. H. Hansen and P. Dombernowsky, p. 161. Excerpta Medica, Amsterdam.

46. Moore, T. N., Livingston, R., Heilburn, L., Eltringham, J., Skinner, O., White, J., and Tesh, D. (1978): The effectiveness of prophylactic brain irradiation in small-cell carcinoma of the lung: A Southwest Oncology Group study. *Cancer*, 41:2,149–2,153.

47. Muggia, F. M., and Rozencweig, M., editors (1979): *Lung cancer: Progress in Therapeutic Research*. Raven Press, New York.

48. Murphy, W. K., Valdivieso, M., Legha, S., and Bodey, G. P. (1980): A phase II study of 4′-9-acridinylamino-methane-sulfon-*m*-anisidide (AMSA) in patients with metastatic lung cancer. *Proc. Am. Assoc. Cancer Res. and ASCO*, 21:456.

49. Myers, J. W., Livingston, R. B., Coltman, C. A., Jr. (1980): Combination chemotherapy of advanced adeno- and large-cell undifferentiated carcinoma of the lung with 5-FU, vincristine, and mitomycin-C (FOMi). *Proc. Am. Assoc. Cancer Res. and ASCO*, 21:453.

50. Natale, R. B., Hilaris, B., Shank, B., and Wittes, R. E. (1980): Prolonged remission of small-cell lung carcinoma (SCLC) with intensive chemotherapy induction and high-dose radiation therapy without maintenance. *Abstracts, II, World Conference on Lung Cancer*, edited by H. H. Hansen and P. Dombernowsky, p. 162. Excerpta Medica, Amsterdam.

51. Nixon, D. W., Murphy, G. F., Sewell, C. W., Kutner, M., and Lynn, M. J. (1979): Relationship between survival and histologic type in small-cell anaplastic carcinoma of the lung. *Cancer*, 44:1,045–1,049.

52. O'Donnell, M., Ruckdeschel, J. C., Sedransk, N., Baxter, D., Spiers, A. S. D., and Horton, J. (1981): Does intensive induction chemotherapy improve survival in small-cell cancer of the lung (SCCL)? A randomized comparison. *Proc. Am. Assoc. Cancer Res. and ASCO*, 22:168.

53. Pazdur, R., Bonomi, P., Lind, M., Rossof, A. H., and Wolter, J. (1980): Phase II trial of mitomycin C (MITO) and hexamethylmelamine (HMM) in metastatic non-oat cell bronchogenic carcinoma (MNOBC). *Proc. Am. Assoc. Cancer Res. and ASCO*, 21:457.

54. Pennachio, J., McBrine, P., Friedman, H., Faling, J., Snider, G., Bhutani, R., and Hong, W. K. (1980): Prospective randomized study of vindesine (DVA) vs DVA with cis-platinum (DDP) in metastatic non-small-cell lung cancer (NSCLC). *Proc. Am. Assoc. Cancer Res. and ASCO*, 21:459.

55. Reynolds, R. E., Frank, J. G., Anson, N. O., Weise, P. B., Grant, D., Donnell, R., Friedman, M. A., Meyers, F., and Carter, S. K. (1980): Phase II trial of M-AMSA in metastatic or recurrent lung cancer. *Proc. Am. Assoc. Cancer Res. and ASCO*, 21:457.

56. Ritter, S. D., Rosenthal, C. J., and Gupta, M. (1980): Bleomycin (B), cis-platinum (C), vincristine (V), and methotrexate (M) combination therapy in advanced carcinoma (CA) of the lung. *Proc. Am. Assoc. Cancer Res. and ASCO*, 21:452.

57. Samson, M. K., Fraile, R. J., Baker, L. H., and Talley, R. W. (1980): A phase II study of AMSA in lung cancer. *Proc. Am. Assoc. Cancer Res. and ASCO*, 21:357.

58. Schabel, F. M., Jr., Trader, M. W., Laster, W. R., Jr., Corbett, T. H., and Griswold, D. P., Jr. (1979): Cis-dichlorodiammineplatinum (II): Combination chemotherapy and cross-resistance studies with tumors of mice. *Cancer Treat. Rep.*, 63:1,459–1,473.

59. Sierocki, J. S., Hilaris, B. S., Hopfan, S., Martini, N., Barton, D., Golbey, R. B., and Wittes, R. E. (1979): Cis-dichlorodiammineplatinum (II) and VP-16-213: An active induction regimen for small-cell carcinoma of the lung. *Cancer Treat. Rep.*, 63:1,593–1,597.

60. Stoopler, M. B., Kelsen, D. P., Gralla, R. J., Casper, E. S., Cheng, E., and Golbey, R. B. (1980): Vindesine (DVA), cis-dichlorodiammineplatinum II (DDP), cytoxan (CTX), and adriamycin (ADR) combination chemotherapy in non-small-cell lung cancer (NSCLC). *Proc. Am. Assoc. Cancer Res. and ASCO*, 21:457.

61. Takita, H., Marabella, P. C., Edgerton, F., and Rizzo, D. (1979): Cis-dichlorodiammineplatinum (II), adriamycin, cyclophosphamide, CCNU, and vincristine in non-small-cell lung carcinoma: A preliminary report. *Cancer Treat. Rep.*, 63:29–33.

62. Van Houtte, P., Tancini, G., De Jager, R., Lustman-Maréchal, J., Milani, F., Bonadonna, G., and Kenis, Y. (1979): Small-cell carcinoma of the lung: A combined modality treatment. *Eur. J. Cancer*, 15:1,159–1,165.

63. Vogl, S. E., and Mehta, C. (1981): Standard (STD) vs intensive (INT) induction chemotherapy of small-cell bronchogenic carcinoma (SCBC) with cyclophosphamide (C), CCNU (Cc), and methotrexate (M), followed by continued CCcM or cyclic maintenance therapy—A randomized trial of the Eastern Cooperative Oncology Group. *Proc. Am. Assoc. Cancer Res. and ASCO*, 22:199.

64. Vogl, S. E., Mehta, C. R., and Cohen, M. H. (1979): MACC chemotherapy for adenocarcinoma and epidermoid carcinoma of the lung: Low response rate in a cooperative group study. *Cancer*, 44:864–868.

65. Vogl, S. E., Wollner, D., Kaplan, B. H., and Berenzweig, M. (1980): Combination chemotherapy for non-small-cell bronchogenic carcinoma with bleomycin, doxorubicin, methotrexate, and cis-dichlorodiammineplatinum (II) (BAMP). *Cancer Treat. Rep.*, 64:717–719.

66. Weissman, C. H., Ruckdeschel, J. C., Reilly, C., and Horton, J. (1980): Cyclophosphamide, adriamycin, and VP-16-213 (CAVP-16) chemotherapy in the management of advanced non-oat cell bronchogenic carcinoma (NOBC). *Proc. Am. Assoc. Cancer Res. and ASCO*, 21:459.

67. Whitehead, R., Crowley, J., and Carbone, P. P. (1980): Cis-dichlorodiammineplatinum (P), adriamycin (A), cyclophosphamide (C), CCNU (C), and vincristine (O) (PACCO) combination chemotherapy in advanced non-small-cell bronchogenic carcinoma. *Proc. Am. Assoc. Cancer Res. and ASCO*, 21:458.

New Approaches in Cancer Therapy,
edited by H. Cortés Funes and M. Rozencweig.
Raven Press, New York © 1982.

Phase II Studies in Non-Small-Cell Lung Cancer: The Memorial Hospital Experience, 1977 to 1980

R. J. Gralla, E. S. Casper, D. P. Kelsen, R. A. Chapman,
L. M. Itri, S. E. Krown, M. B. Stoopler, G. R. Lynch, and
R. B. Golbey

*Developmental Chemotherapy, Solid Tumor and Clinical Immunology Services,
Department of Medicine, Memorial Sloan-Kettering Cancer Center,
Cornell University Medical College, New York, New York 10021*

The investigation of new agents has a high priority in the treatment of patients with non-small-cell lung cancer. Conventional agents, used singly or in combination, have failed to alter significantly the natural history of this malignancy (31). As shown in Table 1, single-agent trials with the more commonly used conventional drugs have been performed in the 1970s. These have not confirmed the high response rates of earlier studies (38). With the recent results considered, several centers have become involved in new drug trials.

This chapter will summarize the results of studies with 10 phase II agents investigated at the Memorial Sloan-Kettering Cancer Center over the past 3 years.

PATIENTS AND METHODS

All patients entered into these trials had objectively measurable disease with histologic or cytologic confirmation of the diagnosis of non-small-cell lung cancer. Patients were required to have a performance status (PS, Karnofsky scale) of ≥ 50, a platelet count $\geq 120,000/mm^2$, and a white blood cell (WBC) count $\geq 4,000/mm^3$.

TABLE 1. *Trials with conventional agents in the 1970s in non-small-cell lung cancer*

Agents	No. of patients	Major response rate (range)		Ref.
Cyclophosphamide	106	10%	(4–13%)	2,14
Methotrexate	130	4.5%	(0–7%)	41
Adriamycin	210	9%	(0–24%)	9,28,29
CCNU[a]	94	10%	(0–31%)	7,26,40

[a]CCNU: 1-(2-chloroethyl)-3-cyclohexyl-L-nitrosourea.

Informed consent was obtained from all patients and pretreatment work-up included: complete history and physical examination, complete blood count, 12-channel biochemical screening profile, 5'-nucleotidase, serum electrolytes and creatinine, prothrombin time, serum glucose, and chest roentgenogram. Liver and bone scans, and computerized transaxial tomography were performed only when clinically indicated. During the trials, patients had weekly or biweekly physical examinations and complete blood counts, biweekly determinations of biochemical tests, and monthly evaluations of chest roentgenograms unless indicated at an earlier date.

Characteristics of the adequately treated patients in each study are listed in Table 2; these include median age, median performance status, and histologic type of tumor. In addition, Table 2 outlines the initial dosage and schedule employed for each agent. Several classes of drugs are represented: alkylating agents {cisplatin and the nitrosoureas chlorozotocin and PCNU[N-(2-chloroethyl)-N-(2,6-dioxo-3-piperidinyl)-N-nitrosourea]}; inhibitors of *de novo* pyrimidine synthesis [phosphonacetyl-L-aspartate (PALA) and pyrazofurin]; a polyamine synthesis inhibitor {methyl GAG[methylglyoxal *bis* (guanylhydrazone)]} an acridine derivative, acridinyl-*m*-sulphoneanisidine (*m*-AMSA); and an immunemodulator (interferon). Adequate treatment required a minimum of one 6-week course with the nitrosoureas; two courses every 3 to 4 weeks with cisplatin, metoprine, or *m*-AMSA; three weekly treatments with vindesine, PALA, pyrazofurin, or methyl GAG; and 1 month of daily i.m. injections of interferon.

Response criteria were defined as: complete remission (CR)—disappearance of all evidence of tumor for $\geqslant 1$ month; partial remission (PR)—$\geqslant 50\%$ decrease of all measurable lesions for $\geqslant 1$ month; minor response (MR)—objective tumor decrease of $>25\%$, but less than that required for a PR; and progression—objective increase in measurable disease, or the appearance of new tumor lesions.

RESULTS

Table 3 outlines the therapeutic results observed during the 10 phase II trials. With six agents, no major responses (CR or PR) were observed. However, with vindesine (22), 22% of patients experienced major responses. By histologic type, responses occurred in 6 of 29 patients with adenocarcinoma, 3 of 14 with epidermoid carcinoma, and 1 of 3 patients with large-cell carcinoma. Median duration of response was 5 months (range, 2 to 9 months).

Four patients, or 10%, experienced PR with methyl GAG given on a weekly schedule. This trial continues to enlist patients, and the median duration of response has not been determined. Responding patients included 2 with epidermoid carcinoma and 2 patients with adenocarcinoma.

With chlorozotocin (6), two major responses were noted among the 30 adequately treated patients. One PR occurred in the high-dose cisplatin trial (7). Of the 19 patients treated with human leukocyte interferon (30), marked increases in natural killer cell activity were observed. However, no objective responses occurred.

The major toxicity observed with seven of the agents was myelosuppression. Of those agents with which little blood count depression was noted, PALA was as-

TABLE 2. *Patient characteristics in phase II trials in non-small-cell lung cancer*

	No. of patients	Median age	Median ps	Percent of patients with:			Dosage and schedule
				Adeno-carcinoma	Epidermoid carcinoma	Large-cell	
Alkylating agents							
Chlorozotocin	30	61	60	60%	37%	3%	150–175 mg/m^2 i.v. q. 6 weeks
PCNU	19	58	60	64%	36%	0%	100–125 mg/m^2 i.v. q. 6 weeks
Cisplatin	18	55	70	50%	33%	17%	120 mg/m^2 i.v. q. 4 weeks
Antimetabolites							
PALA	18	58	70	67%	28%	5%	3.75–4.50 g/m^2 i.v. weekly
Metoprine	24	59	70	83%	17%	0%	50 mg/m^2 p.o. q. 3 weeks
Pyrazofurin	24	58	70	42%	58%	0%	200 mg/m^2 i.v. weekly
Other agents							
Interferon	19	50	70	79%	21%	0%	3.0 × 10^6 units daily × 30 days
m-AMSA	22	61	70	81%	14%	5%	90–120 mg/m^2 i.v. q. 3 weeks
Vindesine	46	59	60	63%	31%	6%	3 mg/m^2 i.v. weekly
Methyl GAG	40	55	70	72%	28%	0%	500 mg/m^2 i.v. weekly

TABLE 3. *Responses in phase II trials in non-small-cell lung cancer*

	No. of patients	CR	PR	MR	Major response rate	Predicted true response rate ($p = 0.05$)	Ref.
Alkylating agents							
Chlorozotocin	30	1	1	4	7%	(2−18%)	6
PCNU	19	0	0	0	0%	(<15%)	23
Cisplatin	18	0	1	2	6%	(<25%)	7
Antimetabolites							
PALA	18	0	0	4	0%	(<16%)	18
Metoprine	24	0	0	1	0%	(<13%)	34
Pyrazofurin	24	0	0	4	0%	(<13%)	21
Other agents							
Interferon	19	0	0	0	0%	(<15%)	30
m-AMSA	22	0	0	1	0%	(<14%)	8
Vindesine	46	0	10	7	22%	(13−35%)	22
Methyl GAG	40	0	4	5	10%	(3−24%)	8a

sociated with dose-limiting gastrointestinal and cutaneous toxicity. In addition to mild myelosuppression, severe emesis and mild nephrotoxicity was observed with cisplatin. On the weekly schedule, no myelosuppression, stomatitis, or hypoglycemia was observed with methyl GAG; however, 20% of patients experienced muscle weakness involving primarily the lower extremities. Among the agents with which moderate myelosuppression was observed, fever with interferon and peripheral neuropathy with vindesine were prominent toxicities.

DISCUSSION

The primary aim of a phase II clinical trial is to determine in a small number of patients if an agent has sufficient activity to warrant further study. Attention to statistical considerations can help to estimate the number of patients needed in a new drug trial (17). In non-small-cell lung cancer, an agent with a greater than 15% predicted true response rate, at 95% confidence limits, deserves further investigation. With the results of the 10 studies outlined in this report, four agents met this criterion for expanded clinical trials.

Cisplatin has now become one of the best-studied new agents in lung cancer in single-drug and combination trials. Clearly, cisplatin in this malignancy does not possess the high degree of activity observed in patients with testicular or ovarian carcinomas (15). However, the overall 14% major response rate in 182 patients (1,3,11,20,36) suggests that it does have a useful role in the treatment of lung cancer. In addition, the relatively mild myelosuppression seen with cisplatin makes it a good candidate for use in combination.

The activity observed with chlorozotocin was similar to that reported with the older nitrosoureas (12,26,40). Combining the results of the trial reported above with those of the study from the Mayo Clinic, an overall 5% major response rate is found in 61 patients (6,10). In this number of patients, the predicted true response rate is less than 15%; with no advantage over the previously tested nitrosoureas, it can be concluded that chlorozotocin is only of marginal value in lung cancer.

Vindesine gave the highest response rate observed in the 10 studies (22). In three recently reported trials with vindesine, similar responses have been seen (16,24,35). Overall 16% and 30% major response rates in squamous and adenocarcinoma, respectively, have been observed in 116 patients. Although no concurrent comparison trials have been performed, vindesine has greater activity than that reported in older studies with vinblastine (32) or vincristine (5,25).

With both vindesine and cisplatin, higher response rates have been observed in patients who have not previously received chemotherapy. As shown in Table 4, this finding has also been seen with methyl GAG, and illustrates that new drug trials should include untreated patients. Methyl GAG, on a weekly administration schedule, has been associated with only mild toxicity and with a 15% response rate in untreated patients. With these findings, further trials with this agent are indicated.

Recently, combinations that have included only newer agents have been studied as initial chemotherapy. Cisplatin has been combined with vindesine and with VP-16-213 [a podophyllin derivative with an 18% major response rate (13)]. In the study using vindesine, two dosage schedules of cisplatin were compared (60 mg/m^2 versus 120 mg/m^2) in a randomized trial (19). Although the response rate, 43%, was similar in both arms of the study, responding patients on the higher-dose cisplatin regimen experienced a longer duration of response (12 months versus 6 months, $p = 0.05$) and improved survival (21.5 months versus 10 months for those responding to low-dose cisplatin, $p = 0.02$). Two ongoing studies using VP-16-213 with cisplatin have reported encouraging response rates of 45% (33) and 33% (27). At present, it is too early to determine survival results for these latter regimens.

Currently, phase II disease-oriented clinical trials are the best way to investigate new drugs. However, newer methods of preclinical testing would help to identify promising agents for clinical studies and could provide a less empirical procedure for the selection of specific drugs for individual patients. Tumor colony assay techniques (4,37) and human tumor xenografts (39) are now being tested at several centers for drug sensitivity and for correlation with clinical response. Results of

TABLE 4. *Effect of prior chemotherapy on response rates in phase II trials in non-small-cell lung cancer*

Agent	No prior chemotherapy		Prior chemotherapy		Ref.
	No. of patients	Major response rate	No. of patients	Major response rate	
Cisplatin	114	19%	68	6%	1,3,7,11,20,36
Vindesine	86	27%	30	13%	16,22,24,35
Methyl GAG	20	15%	20	5%	8a

these and similar trials may help to establish improved methods of new drug investigation.

With the high incidence of lung cancer, and with the likelihood of the disease to be disseminated at initial presentation, the need for improved systemic treatment is obvious. This improvement will require a continued emphasis on the investigation of new agents and on new approaches to lung cancer.

ACKNOWLEDGMENTS

Supported in part by NIH Contract No. 1CM57043 and Grant CA-05826. We wish to thank Kathleen Trainor for preparation of the manuscript.

REFERENCES

1. Berenzweig, M., Vogl, S. E., Kaplan, B. H., et al. (1980): Phase II trial of cis-diamminedichloroplatinum in patients with non-small-cell bronchogenic carcinoma not exposed to prior chemotherapy. *Proc. ASCO and AACR*, 21:457.
2. Bodey, G. P., Lagakos, S. W., Gutierrez, A. C., et al. (1977): Therapy of advanced squamous carcinoma of the lung. *Cancer*, 39:1,026–1,031.
3. Britell, J. C., Eagan, R. T., Ingle, J. N., et al. (1978): Cis-dichlorodiammineplatinum (II) alone followed by adriamycin plus cyclophosphamide at progression versus cis-dichlorodiammineplatinum (II), adriamycin, and cyclophosphamide in combination for adenocarcinoma of the lung. *Cancer Treat. Rep.*, 62:1,207–1,210.
4. Carney, D. N., Gazdar, A. F., and Minna, J. D. (1980): Direct cloning of small-cell carcinoma of the lung. In: *Abstracts on the Second World Conference on Lung Cancer*, edited by H. Hansen and P. Dombernowsky, p. 27. Excerpta Medica, Amsterdam.
5. Brugarolas, A., Lacave, A. J., Ribas, A., et al. (1978): Vincristine (NSC-67574) in non-small-cell bronchogenic carcinoma. Results of a phase II clinical study. *Eur. J. Cancer*, 14:501–505.
6. Casper, E. S., and Gralla, R. J. (1979): Phase II evaluation of chlorozotocin in patients with non-small-cell carcinoma of the lung. *Cancer Treat. Rep.*, 63:549–550.
7. Casper, E. S., Gralla, R. J., Kelsen, D. P., et al. (1979): Phase II study of high-dose cis-diamminedichloroplatinum (II) in the treatment of non-small-cell lung cancer. *Cancer Treat. Rep.*, 63:2,107–2,109.
8. Casper, E. S., Gralla, R. J., Kelsen, D. P., et al. (1981): *m*-AMSA: A phase II evaluation in patients with non-small-cell lung cancer. *Cancer Treat. Rep. (in press)*.
8a. Chapman, R., Kelsen, D., Gralla, R., et al. (1981): Phase II trial of methylglyoxal *bis*(guanylthydrazone) in non-small cell lung cancer. *Cancer Clin. Trials*, 4:389–391.
9. Cortes, E. P., Takita, H., and Holland, J. F. (1974): Adriamycin in advanced bronchogenic carcinoma. *Cancer*, 34:518–525.
10. Creagan, E. T., Eagan, R. T., Fleming, T. R., et al. (1979): Phase II evaluation of chlorozotocin in advanced bronchogenic carcinoma. *Cancer Treat. Rep.*, 63:2,105–2,106.
11. DeJager, R., Libert, P., Michel, J., et al. (1980): Phase II clinical trials with high-dose cisplatin with mannitol-induced diuresis in advanced bronchogenic cancer. *Proc. ASCO and AACR*, 21:363.
12. Eagan, R. T., Carr, D. T., Coles, D. T., et al. (1974): Randomized study comparing CCNU and methyl CCNU in advanced bronchogenic carcinoma. *Cancer Chemother. Rep.*, 58:913–918.
13. Eagan, R. T., Ingle, J. N., Creagan, E. T., et al. (1978): VP-16-213 chemotherapy for advanced squamous cell carcinoma and adenocarcinoma of the lung. *Cancer Treat. Rep.*, 62:843–844.
14. Edmonson, J. H., Lagakos, S. W., Selawry, O. S., et al. (1976): Cyclophosphamide and CCNU in the treatment of inoperable small-cell carcinoma and adenocarcinoma of the lung. *Cancer Treat. Rep.*, 60:925–932.
15. Einhorn, L. H., and Williams, S. D. (1979): The role of cis-platinum in solid tumor therapy. *N. Engl. J. Med.*, 300:289–291.
16. Furnas, B., Einhorn, L. H., and Rohn, R. J. (1980): A phase II trial of vindesine in non-small-cell lung cancer. *Proc. ASCO and AACR*, 21:48.
17. Gehan, E. A. (1961): The determination of the number of patients required in a preliminary and a follow-up trial of a new chemotherapeutic agent. *J. Chronic Dis.*, 13:346–353.

18. Gralla, R. J., Casper, E. S., and Golbey, R. B. (1979): Phase I and preliminary phase II studies with N-(phosphonacetyl)-L-aspartic acid (PALA). *Proc. ASCO and AACR*, 20:115.
19. Gralla, R. J., Casper, E. S., Kelsen, D. P., et al. (1981): Cisplatin vindesine combination chemotherapy for advanced carcinoma of the lung: A randomized trial investigating two dosage schedules. *Ann. Int. Med.*, 95:414–420.
20. Gralla, R. J., Cvitkovic, E., and Golbey, R. B. (1979): Cis-dichlorodiammineplatinum (II) in non-small-cell carcinoma of the lung. *Cancer Treat. Rep.*, 63:1,585–1,588.
21. Gralla, R. J., Currie, V. E., Wittes, R. E., et al. (1978): Phase II evaluation of pyrazofurin in patients with carcinoma of the lung. *Cancer Treat. Rep.*, 62:451–452.
22. Gralla, R. J., Raphael, B. G., Golbey, R. B., et al. (1979): Phase II evaluation of vindesine in patients with non-small-cell carcinoma of the lung. *Cancer Treat. Rep.*, 63:1,343–1,346.
23. Gralla, R. J., Young, C. W., Tan, C. T., et al. (1980): Phase I study of PCNU. *Proc. ASCO and AACR*, 21:185.
24. Grundtvig, P., Osterlind, K., Pedersen, A. G., et al. (1980): Phase II trial of vindesine in bronchogenic carcinoma of W.H.O. types I, III, and IV. In: *Abstracts of the Second World Conference on Lung Cancer*, edited by H. Hansen and P. Dombernowsky, p. 230. Excerpta Medica, Amsterdam.
25. Holland, J. F., Scharlau, C., Gailani, S., et al. (1973): Vincristine treatment of advanced cancer: A cooperative study of 392 cases. *Cancer Res.*, 33:1,258–1,264.
26. Hoogstraten, B., Gottlieb, J. A., Caoili, E., et al. (1973): CCNU (1-(2-chloroethyl)-3-cyclohexyl-*l*-nitrosourea) in the treatment of cancer—Phase II study. *Cancer*, 32:38–43.
27. Joss, R., Goldhirsch, Cavalli, F., et al. (1980): Cis-platinum and VP-16-213 combination chemotherapy for non-small-cell lung cancer. In: *Abstracts of the Second World Conference on Lung Cancer*, edited by H. Hansen and P. Dombernowsky, p. 233. Excerpta Medica, Amsterdam.
28. Krakoff, I. H. (1975): Adriamycin (NSC-123127) studies in adult patients. *Cancer Chemother. Rep.*, 6:253–257.
29. Knight, E. W., Lagakos, S., Stolbach, L., et al. (1976): Adriamycin in the treatment of far-advanced lung cancer. *Cancer Treat. Rep.*, 60:939–941.
30. Krown, S. E., Stoopler, M. B., Gralla, R. J., et al. (1982): Phase II trial of human leukocyte interferon in non-small-cell lung cancer—Preliminary results. In: *Immunotherapy of Human Cancer*, edited by W. D. Terry and S. Rosenberg. Elsevier/North-Holland, New York.
31. Livingston, R. B. (1977): Combination chemotherapy of bronchogenic carcinoma. I. Non-oat cell. *Cancer Treat. Rep.*, 4:153–165.
32. Livingston, R. B., and Carter, S. K. (1970): *Single Agents in Cancer Chemotherapy*, pp. 279–297. IFI/Plenum, New York, New York.
33. Longeval, E., DeJager, R., Tagnon, H., et al. (1980): Cisplatin-VP-16-213 combination chemotherapy in non-small-cell bronchogenic carcinoma: Phase I–II clinical trial. *Proc. ASCO and AACR*, 21:368.
34. Lynch, G., Kemeny, N., Gralla, R., et al. (1980): Phase II trials of metoprine in patients with colorectal carcinoma and non-small-cell lung carcinoma. *Proc. ASCO and AACR*, 21:351.
35. Pennachio, J., McBrine, P., Friedman, H., et al. (1980): Prospective randomized study of vindesine (DVA) vs. DVA with cisplatinum in metastatic non-small-cell lung cancer. *Proc. ASCO and AACR*, 21:459.
36. Rossof, A. H., Bearden, J. D., and Coltman, C. A. (1976): Phase II evaluation of cis-diamminedichloroplatinum (II) in lung cancer. *Cancer Treat. Rep.*, 60:1,679–1,680.
37. Salmon, S. E., Hamburger, A. W., Soehnlen, B., et al. (1978): Quantitation of differential sensitivity of human tumor stem cells to anticancer drugs. *N. Engl. J. Med.*, 298:1,321–1,327.
38. Selawry, O. S. (1973): Monochemotherapy of bronchogenic carcinoma with special reference to cell type. *Cancer Chemother. Rep.*, 4:177–188.
39. Shorthouse, A. J., Smyth, J. F., Peckham, M. J. (1980): Comparison of the chemosensitivity of bronchial carcinoma xenografts with donor patients. *Proc. ASCO and AACR*, 21:447.
40. Takita, H., and Brugarolas, A. (1973): Effect of CCNU (NSC-79037) on bronchogenic carcinoma. *J. Natl. Cancer Inst.*, 50:49–53.
41. Vincent, R. G., Pickren, J. W., Fergen, T. B., et al. (1975): Evaluation of methotrexate in the treatment of bronchogenic carcinoma. *Cancer*, 36:873–880.

New Approaches in Cancer Therapy,
edited by H. Cortés Funes and M. Rozencweig.
Raven Press, New York © 1982.

Chemotherapy of Adult Soft Tissue Sarcomas

*V. H. C. Bramwell, **G. Stoter, and †H. M. Pinedo

*Cancer Research Campaign, Department of Medical Oncology, Manchester University
and Christie Hospital and Holt Radium Institute, United Kingdom; **Free University
Hospital; and †Netherlands Cancer Institute, Amsterdam, The Netherlands

CHEMOTHERAPY FOR ADVANCED DISEASE

We will discuss both single agents and combination regimens that have shown activity in advanced soft tissue sarcoma. In contrast with the sensitivity of childhood sarcomas to vincristine, cyclophosphamide, and actinomycin D, there has been no evidence for activity of these drugs as single agents in advanced adult soft tissue sarcomas. For this reason they will not be mentioned in the following paragraphs.

Single-Agent Chemotherapy and Analogs

Adriamycin

Adriamycin is the most effective agent in adult soft tissue sarcoma, reported responses ranging from 9 to 79%, depending on prior chemotherapy, dose, scheduling, and the number of patients in the various studies (21). Several investigators have reexamined adriamycin as a single agent. A variety of dosages and schedules have been studied (Table 1). Creagan et al. (8) have treated 15 patients with 20 to 25 mg/m² three times daily every 3 weeks. There was 1 objective response lasting 6 weeks and 8 patients had stable disease for 3 to 4 months. Rosenbaum and Schoenfeld (30), who compared adriamycin with combination chemotherapy, treated 39 patients with 70 mg/m² adriamycin every 3 weeks, and obtained 3 complete remissions and 8 partial remissions, a total response rate of 28%. This confirms the findings of others that adriamycin is best given as a single large dose every 3 to 4 weeks. The Central Oncology Group also confirmed the 30 to 40% response rate reported in the literature for adriamycin in soft tissue sarcoma (19). The second study (7) by this group had poorer results, possibly because of the less intensive schedule; if patients with prior chemotherapy are excluded, however, the response rate rises to 22%. The response rate of 6% for uterine sarcomas reported by Piver and Barlow (27) is very low, in contrast to the 27.5% response rate in 51 patients

TABLE 1. *Different dosages and schedules of adriamycin in soft tissue sarcomas*

Dosage	No. evaluable	CR N(%)	PR N(%)	CR + PR (%)	Ref.
0.4 mg/kg, days 1–3, 8–10, then 0.4 mg/kg/wk	36[a]	3(8)	11(31)	39	20
1 mg/kg/wk until toxicity, then 0.5 mg/kg/wk	35[a]	3(9)	6(17)	26	5
0.4 mg/kg, days 1–3, 8–10, then every 2 wks starting day 15	41[b]	1(2)	6(15)	7	8
60 mg/m^2 every 3 wks	63[c]	2(3)	6(10)	13	33
70 mg/m^2 every 3 wks	39[d]	3(8)	8(20)	28	30
90 mg/m^2 every 3 wks	17[a]	0	1(6)	6	27
20–25 mg/m^2, days 1–3, every 3 wks	15[c]	0	1(6)	6	7

[a]Not specified if patients received prior chemotherapy—the majority probably did not.
[b]14 received prior chemotherapy.
[c]Most received prior chemotherapy.
[d]None had prior chemotherapy.

reported by Omura and Blessing (22). Unfortunately, Piver and Barlow do not analyse response according to histological subtype, which may be an important prognostic variable in uterine sarcomas. If the study included a large proportion of mixed mesodermal tumors, the poor response rate would be less surprising.

Analogs of adriamycin are of considerable interest, as adriamycin is the single most active drug in soft tissue sarcoma. Carminomycin is the only one that has been tested in the past with a 27% response rate in 48 patients (23). However, in a large randomized phase II study recently performed by the EORTC Soft Tissue and Bone Sarcoma Group, in which the effect of adriamycin was compared with that of carminomycin, the results with the latter were disappointing. This group is presently performing a similar randomized study in which carminomycin has been replaced by 4'epiadriamycin. In addition, aclacinomycin A, AD32, detorubicin, quelamycin, and rubidazone are being studied by other groups (35).

Methotrexate

Subramanian and Wiltshaw (36) have reported 75 patients treated with methotrexate alone or in combination. Forty-one patients received low- or medium-dose methotrexate. There were 6 complete remissions and 9 partial remissions—an overall response rate of 36%. Three different dosage regimens—(a) oral 2.5 to 10 mg daily for 2 to 15 days; (b) i.v. 50 to 100 mg every 2 to 3 weeks or 50 to 500 mg infusion over 18 to 36 hr every 4 weeks; (c) i.a. 50 mg in 24 hr for 4 days—were used, and it is not clear from the report which was the most effective. An interesting observation was that those patients with metastatic disease had an inferior response rate to those with inoperable or locally recurrent tumor (26 versus 57%).

Karakousis (13) described 3 complete remissions, 2 lasting 3 months, the other continuing at 8 months, in 13 patients relapsing from the combination of cyclophosphamide, vincristine, adriamycin, and dacarbazine (CYVADIC) treated with 4 g/m² methotrexate followed by folinic acid (Leucovorin) rescue. More recently, the same author reported only 1 remission in 18 patients who received the same dose of methotrexate (14). Isacoff et al. (12), using escalating doses of methotrexate from 50 to 300 mg/kg, reported 5 partial remissions in 11 patients with soft tissue sarcoma.

At present, there is no evidence that high-dose methotrexate has any advantage over low or medium doses of the drug in soft tissue sarcoma.

Other Drugs Recently Investigated

The lack of response of soft tissue sarcomas to cisplatin in the study reported by the EORTC (3,4) is in contrast to the activity of this drug in osteosarcoma. Most of the other drugs which have been studied recently, such as lomustine (CCNU), acridinyl-*m*-sulphone anisidine (AMSA), chlorozotocin, pyrazofurin, dibromodulcitol, maytansine, cycloleucine, piperazinedione, and 5-azacytidine, appear to be inactive (6,19,20,35,36). Razoxane may be active in enhancing radiation damage to soft tissue sarcomas (11). Some activity has been observed with vindesine (19).

Combination Chemotherapy

CYVADIC combination used by the SWOG still has the highest reported response rate (55%) in soft tissue sarcoma (10). However, in a recent reevaluation, the response rate in a similar group of patients was somewhat lower (50%) (38). The randomized study of Rodriguez et al. (29) that confirmed the efficacy of this combination also suggested that dose escalation might improve response rate, although no prolongation of survival was observed.

In contrast to the SWOG study of CYVADIC in which a response rate as high as 59% was recorded for soft tissue sarcomas (24), the EORTC (25), in their randomized protocol comparing two schedules of the same drugs, found a 37% response rate despite only minimal modification of the classic schedule (Table 2). Doses were similar to those in the SWOG study, but the drugs were administered every 4 weeks in the EORTC study. Patients in the cycling arm of the trial received pairs of drugs [cyclophosphamide/vincristine and adriamycin/dacarbazine (DTIC)] alternating at 4-weekly intervals. The difference in response rate between the full (37%) and the split regimen (23%) is significant ($p < 0.05$).

Recently, the combination of cyclophosphamide, adriamycin, and DTIC has given a 56% response rate in 23 patients (2). Although this figure is interesting, the number of patients needs to be expanded.

Other Combinations Recently Investigated

A 36% response rate has been achieved (17) in 100 evaluable patients using the combination of adriamycin, cyclophosphamide, and methotrexate (ACM). Median survival (11 months) was the same for responders and nonresponders.

TABLE 2. Combinations including adriamycin

Combination	No. of evaluable patients	No. of respond.			Response rate (%)			Ref.
		CR	PR	Overall	CR	PR	Overall	
ADM/DTIC							22	
ADM/DTIC/CTX	243						35	2
ADM/DTIC/ACD							25	
ADM/DTIC/CTX	23	4	9	13	17	39	56	3
CTX/VCR/ADM/DTIC(CYVADIC)	119	19	41	60	16	34	50	39
CTX/VCR/ADM/DTIC(CYVADIC)	60	8	14	22	13	23	37	25
VCR(SPLIT CYVADIC)/DTIC+CTX/ADM	52	3	9	12	6	17	23	
CTX/VCR/HDMTX-CF/DTIC/ADM(CYOMAD)	38	4	6	10	11	16	27	18
ADM/ACD	21	2	4	6	10	19	29	
ADM/DTIC/HDMTX-CF(STS-1)	23	5	6	11	22	26	48	
ADM/VCR/ACD/CTX/HDMTX-CF(STS II)	40	2	9	11	5	23	28	35–37
ADM/CTX/VCR/LDMTX(STS III)	11	1	3	4	9	27	36	
ADM/CTX/CDDP	20	1	4	5	4	16	20	
ADM/MeCCNU	41	3	17	20	7.5	41.5	49	28

Abbreviations: ADM, adriamycin; CTX, cyclophosphamide; ACD, actinomycin D; VCR, vincristine; MTX, methotrexate; HDMTX, high-dose MTX; LDMTX, low-dose MTX; CDDP, cisplatin.

The study reported by Subramanian and Wiltshaw (36) comparing methotrexate alone with the combination of vincristine, cyclophosphamide, actinomycin D, methotrexate and 5-fluorouracil and that of adriamycin, DTIC, and methotrexate showed a 43% overall response rate in 75 patients, with 12 patients achieving a complete remission. Those with localized disease seemed more likely to respond (49%, with 23% complete remissions) than those with pulmonary metastases or widespread dissemination (36%, with 5% complete remissions). The authors concluded that they could find no evidence that their combination chemotherapy gave better response rates than methotrexate alone.

Rosenbaum and Schoenfeld (30) have reported a randomized study carried out by the Eastern Oncology Group comparing adriamycin with adriamycin/cyclophosphamide/vincristine and vincristine/actinomycin D/cyclophosphamide (VAC), response rates being 28%, 13%, and 5%, respectively, with approximately 38 patients in each arm. This confirms earlier studies indicating that combinations containing actinomycin D, particularly VAC, have little activity in adult sarcomas. The poor response for the combination including adriamycin is surprising.

Memorial Sloan Kettering (18) combined their most effective regime—vincristine (Oncovin®), methotrexate, adriamycin (OMAD)—with CYVADIC to form CY-OMAD. Perhaps not surprisingly, the combination was much more toxic than either regimen alone and probably less active (27% response in 38 patients). Indeed, similar responses might be expected from adriamycin alone.

The Central Oncology Group (8,20) has used a series of single agents and combinations, which, with the exception of adriamycin, seem to have little activity in soft tissue sarcoma.

The analysis by Yap (39) of 53 patients, treated at the M. D. Anderson Hospital, who achieved complete remission on adriamycin-containing regimens, provides some guidelines for future studies. All patients had a minimum follow-up of 18 months. Fifteen patients had advanced local disease and their median duration of remission and survival (23 and 39 months, respectively) were significantly longer than the corresponding values for 38 patients with distant metastases (11 and 27 months). Twenty-three percent of patients remained in continuous remission for a median duration of 37+ months (range, 20 to 53+). Forty-one patients had relapsed, 63% at the original site of disease, 27% at a new site, and 10% combined. Eight patients with locally advanced disease and 5 with distant metastases achieved a partial remission that was converted to a complete remission by surgery. Their median duration of remission was 19.5 months and of survival was 44 months (again longer for locally advanced disease), which were better than for partial remission alone and compared favorably with complete remission. Thus, administration of chemotherapy to patients with advanced local disease seems particularly worthwhile, as complete remissions may be long lasting and partial remissions may be subsequently amenable to surgery with equally good results.

It is possible that uterine sarcomas may be less responsive to chemotherapy than other soft tissue sarcomas. A 27.5% response rate has been reported (22) in 91 patients treated with adriamycin alone (14 of 51 patients) or in combination with

DTIC (11 of 40 patients). The median duration of response was similar for the two regimens (4.2 months and 5.3 months, respectively). It was also noted that leiomyosarcoma appeared to be more responsive than heterologous mixed mesodermal sarcoma.

ADJUVANT CHEMOTHERAPY IN SOFT TISSUE SARCOMA

Although generally less aggressive than osteosarcomas, soft tissue sarcomas are often treated inadequately and have a high rate of local recurrence and ultimate dissemination. The more indolent nature of many of these tumors and the lack of adequate chemotherapy for metastatic disease have meant that there has been little interest in the subject, apart from sporadic reports of uncontrolled series that often use isolated limb perfusion techniques. Reports of adjuvant therapy are limited to two important studies. The first one (32) is a randomized study comparing amputation of the extremity with limb-sparing surgery and postoperative radiotherapy, both groups receiving adjuvant chemotherapy (adriamycin: HDMCTX-CF/cyclophosphamide) $\pm$ immunotherapy ($C. parvum$). The value of adjuvant chemotherapy was assessed by comparison with a historical control group of 66 patients treated at the NCI by radical surgery alone. For extremity tumors there had been 8 relapses in 26 patients, 2 local and 6 with distant metastases. There was no statistical difference in disease-free interval and survival between the three treatment groups, although the 2 local recurrences occurred in patients having conservative surgery. For tumors of the head, neck, and trunk, there had been 6 relapses in 23 patients, 2 local and 4 with distant metastases, with no differences between the two treatment groups. Thus, in the 49 protocol patients, there had been 14 relapses and 7 deaths, with a median follow-up of 38 months (range, 27 to 52 months) compared with 36 relapses and 29 deaths in the 66 historical controls. Actuarial analysis showed a significant improvement in disease-free interval ($p < 0.01$) and survival ($p < 0.01$) for protocol patients, although it is interesting to note that in the previous analysis (36), at a median of 16 months follow-up, the significance level for both these parameters was much higher ($p < 0.001$). One hopes that these curves do not continue to converge with the further passage of time. The addition of immunotherapy to chemotherapy conferred no significant advantage.

The problems associated with the use of historical controls have been recognized by the coordinators of this study and the NCI's current adjuvant sarcoma protocol randomizes patients with extremity tumors between amputation with chemotherapy, limb-sparing surgery with radiotherapy and chemotherapy, and limb-sparing surgery with radiotherapy alone. Patients with sarcoma of the head, neck, or trunk are randomized between surgery plus radiotherapy and surgery with both radiation and chemotherapy.

The second study reported (34) uses a complex regimen of vincristine[HDMTX-CF/adriamycin/DTIC/chlorambucil/actinomycin D(ALOMAD)] given over approximately 10 weeks following surgery. An initial large group of 61 evaluable patients was broken down into five subgroups. Group 1 consisted of 19 patients given adjuvant therapy following removal of a primary tumor; there had been 1 local recurrence, with 18 patients having no evidence of disease 3 to 34 months (median, 15) from surgery. Group 2 comprised 8 patients treated for locally recurrent tumor; there had been 1 local recurrence and 1 patient had developed distant metastases, with the rest having no evidence of disease 4 to 33 months (median, 16) from surgery. The remaining three groups included patients given postoperative radiotherapy because of inadequate surgical margins (group 3), preoperative radiotherapy and adriamycin for large tumors (group 4), and chemotherapy administered after resection of pulmonary metastases (group 5). Taking these three groups together, there had been 13 recurrences in 34 patients. No proper assessment of the value of adjuvant chemotherapy can be made from this study because of the small numbers of patients, lack of a concurrent untreated control group, and short follow-up. It should be noted that ALOMAD has been shown to be relatively ineffective in advanced soft tissue sarcoma (27% response rate in 33 patients) (20).

The adjuvant protocol of the EORTC study has recently been published (26). The aim of this multicenter collaborative trial is to establish if CYVADIC chemotherapy, known to be effective in metastatic disease, can reduce local and distant recurrences and improve survival in patients who have had adequate local surgery. All macroscopic tumor must be resected, although microscopic residual disease is permitted. These latter cases, those with less than 1-cm tumor-free margins around the histological specimen and those who have had a local recurrence, receive postoperative radiotherapy. On completion of surgery and radiotherapy, not more than 13 weeks from the first operation, patients are randomized into a control group receiving no further treatment or a chemotherapy group receiving eight 3-day courses of CYVADIC at monthly intervals. Approximately 60 patients were entered in the 1st year of the study, and it is estimated that 200 eligible patients will be required to provide a reliable answer. Both the new NCI study and the EORTC study will take time to accrue patients with this rare tumor. Adequate duration of follow-up is essential, because late relapse may occur.

REGIONAL PERFUSION AND COMBINED MODALITY TREATMENT

Local recurrence is a significant problem in soft tissue sarcoma, and over the years there have been many studies examining the value of regional perfusion with cytotoxic agents for limb sarcomas, usually as an adjunct to surgery. Studies in dogs (9) and humans (15) have shown that isolation perfusion with adriamycin, using a tourniquet to isolate the limb, will result in 10-fold higher levels of adriamycin in skin, subcutaneous, muscle, and nerve tissue of the perfused limb, with no adriamycin detectable in the nonperfused extremity and minimal systemic blood levels. However, one of the main problems of this technique is a high rate of local toxicity, which is evident from a report by Krementz et al. (15) of 123 perfusions in 113 patients. Complications, sometimes multiple, occurred in 39 patients. These included 9 with wound complications (infections, bleeding, herniation), 30 with tissue damage (skin, nerve, muscle), 15 with systemic problems (hepatic and renal failure, cardiac arrhythmias, pneumonia, and emboli) and 20 with bone marrow depression. Three deaths occurred in the first 6 weeks and 3 patients required amputation for complications of perfusion. Drugs used were melphalan alone (40 patients), mustine alone (39 patients), a combination of melphalan and actinomycin D (20 patients), and other drugs (5-fluorouracil, thiotepa, adriamycin). This study covered the years 1957 to 1975; the authors noted that fewer complications occurred with increasing experience and refinement of the technique, which included the use of an oxygenator in the perfusion apparatus and the introduction of hyperthermia. The response to perfusion alone could be evaluated in 54 patients and was as high as 83%, but only 4 had a complete regression of the tumor lasting more than 3 months. When perfusion was followed by immediate wide excision, the 5-year survival was 66% for 49 localized tumors and 59% for 24 locally recurrent tumors or extensive regional disease including nodes. However, it is possible that similar results could have been obtained by surgery alone, although more amputations may have been necessary. In 9 of 18 patients with inoperable tumors, palliation of pain was achieved, and in 10 of 17 patients, an inoperable tumor shrank sufficiently to allow wide local excision. It should be noted that this group of 113 patients included 11 osteosarcomas (2 paraosteal), 4 chondrosarcomas, 1 Ewing's sarcoma, 3 desmoids, and 5 lymphomas.

As in trials of systemic adjuvant chemotherapy, the lack of a concurrent control group and the heterogeneity of tumors treated make evaluation of the role of limb perfusion with cytotoxic drugs difficult. Certainly, the toxicity of the technique means that it should only be applied in experienced centers, which limits its usefulness.

Lokich (16) advocates combined modality therapy, emphasizing preoperative chemotherapy, although more data are needed to support this. Bearing in mind the encouraging results obtained by Rosen in osteosarcoma, the concept of preoperative systemic combination chemotherapy is attractive, as it may determine the sensitivity of the tumor to chemotherapy, eliminate micrometastases at an early stage, and possibly render an initially inoperable tumor surgically resectable without the use of i.a. vesicant drugs.

However, in contrast to osteosarcomas, most of which are high-grade tumors, there may be considerable differences between the response to chemotherapy of bulky, low- or intermediate-grade, primary soft tissue sarcomas and their systemic micrometastases. It is well known that there may be marked variation in mitotic activity in different areas of the primary tumor, and experience with advanced local and metastatic disease in the same patient has shown that it is possible to get progression of the primary tumor with regression of metastases or vice-versa.

CONCLUSION

Adriamycin forms the backbone of combination chemotherapy for soft tissue sarcomas. The addition of DTIC, vincristine, and cyclophosphamide increases the therapeutic effect to a limited extent. The cycling CYVADIC regimen of EORTC gave a lower response rate, but the duration of response was similar to that seen in the conventional CYVADIC. As adriamycin may be discontinued due to fear of cardiotoxicity, with consequent relapse of responding patients, there is a great need for phase II studies with new anthracyclines. It is preferable that phase II studies are not performed in extensively pretreated patients, as effective agents may be missed.

The development of an effective adjuvant chemotherapeutic regimen may circumvent the problem of lack of antitumor effect of cytotoxic drugs due to high bulk in advanced disease.

REFERENCES

1. Baker, L., Benjamin, R., Fine, G., Saiki, J., and Rivkin, S. (1979): Combination chemotherapy in the management of disseminated soft tissue sarcomas. A Southwest Oncology Group (SWOG) study. *Proc. Am. Soc. Clin. Oncol.*, 20:378.
2. Blum, R. M., Corson, H. J. M., Wilson, R. E., Greenberger, J., Canellos, G. P., and Frei, E. (1980): Successful treatment of metastatic sarcomas with cyclophosphamide, adriamycin, and DTIC. *Cancer*, 46:1,722.
3. Bramwell, V. H. C., Brugarolas, A., Mouridsen, H. T., Cheix, F., De Jager, E., Van Oosterom, A. T., Vendrik, C. P. J., Pinedo, H. M., Sylvester, R., and De Pauw, M. (1979): EORTC phase II study of cisplatin in cyvadic-resistant soft tissue sarcoma. *Eur. J. Cancer*, 15:1,511–1,513.
4. Bramwell, V. H. C., and Pinedo, H. M. (1981): Bone and soft tissue sarcomas. In: *The EORTC Cancer Chemotherapy Annual 3*, edited by H. M. Pinedo. Excerpta Medica, Amsterdam *(in press)*.
5. Chlebowski, R. T., Paroly, W. S., Pugh, R. P., Hueser, J., Jacobs, E. M., Pajak, T. F., and Bateman, J. R. (1980): Adriamycin given as a weekly schedule without a loading course: Clinically effective with reduced incidence of cardiotoxicity. *Cancer Treat. Rep.*, 64:47–51.
6. Cormier, W. J., Hahn, R. G., Edmonson, J. H., and Eagan, R. T. (1980): Phase II study of advanced sarcoma: Randomised trial of pyrazofurin versus combination of cyclophosphamide, doxorubicin, and cis-dichlorodiammineplatinum II (CAP). *Cancer Treat. Rep.*, 64:655.
7. Creagan, E. T., Hahn, R. G., Ahmann, D. L., and Bisel, H. F. (1977): A clinical trial with adriamycin (NSC-123127) in advanced sarcomas. *Oncology*, 34:90–91.
8. Cruz, A. B., Thames, E. A., Aust, J. B., Metter, G., Ramirez, G., Fletcher, W. S., Altman, S. J., and Frelick, R. W. (1979): Combination chemotherapy for soft tissue sarcomas: A phase III study. *J. Surg. Oncol.*, 11:313–323.
9. Didolkar, M. S., Kanter, P. M., Baffi, R. R., Schwartz, H. S., Lopez, R., and Baez, N. (1978): Comparison of regional versus systemic chemotherapy with adriamycin. *Ann. Surg.*, 187:332–336.
10. Gottlieb, J. A., Baker, L. M., O'Bryan, R. M., Sinkovics, J. G., Hoogstraten, B., Quagliana, J. M., Rivkin, S. E., Bodey, G. P., Rodriquez, V. T., Blumenschein, G. R., Jaiki, J. H., Coltman, C., Burgess, M. A., Sullivan, P., Thigpen, T., Bottomley, R., Balcerzak, S., and Moon, T. E. (1975): Adriamycin (NSC-123127) used alone and in combination for soft tissue sarcomas. *Cancer Chemother. Rep.*, 6:271–282.
11. Hellman, K., Ryall, R. D. H., MacDonald, E. K., Newton, K. A., James, S. E., and Jones, S. (1978): Comparison of radiotherapy with and without razoxane (ICRF-159) in the treatment of soft tissue sarcomas. *Cancer*, 41:100–107.
12. Isacoff, W. H., Eilber, F., Cowe, L., Dollinger, M., Lemkin, S., Sheehy, P., Rosenbloom, B., Tabbarah, H., Klein, P., and Block, J. B. (1978): A Phase II clinical trial with high-dose methotrexate therapy and leucovorin rescue. *Cancer Treat. Rep.*, 62:1,295–1,304.
13. Karakousis, C. P. (1978): High-dose methotrexate in metastatic sarcomas. *Proc. Am. Soc. Clin. Oncol.*, 19:401.
14. Karakousis, C. P. (1980): High-dose methotrexate as secondary chemotherapy in metastatic soft tissue sarcoma. *Cancer*, 46:1,345.
15. Krementz, E. T., Carter, R. D., Sutherland, C. M., and Hutton, I. (1977): Chemotherapy of sarcomas of the limbs by regional perfusion. *Ann. Surg.*, 185:555–564.
16. Lokich, J. J. (1979): Preoperative chemotherapy in soft tissue sarcoma. *Surg. Gynecol. Obstet.*, 148:512–516.

17. Lowenbraun, S., Moffit, S., Smalley, R., and Presant, C. (1977): Combination chemotherapy with adriamycin, cyclophosphamide, and methotrexate (ACM) in metastatic sarcomas. *Proc. Am. Soc. Clin. Oncol.*, 18:186.
18. Lynch, G., Magill, G. B., and Golbey, R. B. (1979): Combination chemotherapy of soft part sarcomas with CYOMAD (S-7). *Proc. Am. Assoc. Cancer Res.*, 20:116.
19. Magill, G. B., Golbey, R. B., and Krakoff, I. H. (1977): Chemotherapy combinations in adult sarcomas. *Proc. Am. Soc. Clin. Oncol.*, 18:332.
20. Mitts, D. L., Gerhardt, H., Armstrong, D., Aust, J. B., and Cruz, A. B. (1979): Chemotherapy for advanced soft tissue sarcomas: Results of Phase I and II cooperative studies. *Tex. Med.*, 75:43–47.
21. O'Bryan, R. M., Luce, J. K., Talley, R. W., Gottlieb, J. A., Baker, L. H., and Bonadonna, G. (1973): Phase II evaluation of adriamycin in human neoplasia. *Cancer*, 32:1–8.
22. Omura, G. A., and Blessing, J. A. (1978): Chemotherapy of stage III, IV and recurrent uterine sarcomas: A randomized trial of adriamycin versus adriamycin + dimethyltriazino carboxamide. *Proc. Am. Assoc. Cancer Res.*, 19:26.
23. Perevodchikova, N. I., Lichnitser, M. R., and Gorbunova, V. A. (1977): Phase I clinical study of carminomycin: Its activity against soft tissue sarcomas. *Cancer Treat. Rep.*, 61:1,705–1,707.
24. Pinedo, H. M., and Kenis, Y. (1977): Chemotherapy of advanced soft tissue sarcoma in adults. *Cancer Treat. Rev.*, 4:67–86.
25. Pinedo, H. M., Vendrik, C. P. J., Bramwell, V. H. C., Mouridsen, H. T., Somers, R., Van Oosterom, A. T., Wagener, T., Lewis, B. J., De Pauw, M., Sylvester, R., and Bonadonna, G. (1979): Reevaluation of the CYVADIC regimen for metastatic soft tissue sarcoma. *Proc. Am. Soc. Clin. Oncol.*, 20:346.
26. Pinedo, H. M., Vendrik, C. P. J., Bramwell, V. H. C., Van Slooten, E. A., Deakin, D. P., Van Unnik, J. A. M., Staquet, M., Sylvester, R., and Bonadonna, G. (1979): Evaluation of adjuvant therapy in soft tissue sarcoma: A collaborative multidisciplinary approach (EORTC protocol, 62771). *Eur. J. Cancer*, 15:811–820.
27. Piver, M. S., and Barlow, J. J. (1979): Adriamycin in localised and metastatic uterine sarcoma. *J. Surg. Oncol.*, 12:263.
28. Rivkin, S., Gottlieb, J. A., Thigpen, M. T., El Mawla, N. G., Saiki, J., and Dixon, D. O. (1980): Methyl CCNU and adriamycin for patients with metastatic sarcomas. A Southwest Oncology Group Study. *Cancer*, 44:446.
29. Rodriguez, V., Bodey, C. P., and Freireich, E. J. (1977): Increased remission rate and prolongation of survival in patients with soft tissue sarcomas treated with intensive chemotherapy on a protected environment-prophylactic antibiotic programme (PEPA). *Proc. Am. Soc. Clin. Oncol.*, 18:320.
30. Rosenbaum, C., and Schoenfeld, D. (1977): Treatment of advanced soft tissue sarcoma. *Proc. Am. Soc. Clin. Oncol.*, 18:287.
31. Rosenberg, S. A., Kent, H., Costa, J., Weber, B. L., Young, R., Chabner, B., Baker, A. T., Bremman, M. F., Chretien, P. B., Cohen, M. H., Demoss, E. V., Sears, H. F., Seiff, C., and Simon, R. (1978): Prospective evaluation of the role of limb-sparing surgery, radiation therapy, and adjuvant chemotherapy in the treatment of adult soft tissue sarcomas. *Surgery*, 84:62–69.
32. Rosenberg, S. A., and Sindelar, W. F. (1980): Surgery and adjuvant radiation- and chemo-immunotherapy in soft tissue sarcomas: Results of treatment at the National Cancer Institute. In: *International Course on Recent Advances in the Treatment of Ovarian and Testicular Cancer and of Soft Tissue and Bone Sarcomas*, edited by A. T. Van Oosterom, F. M. Muggia, and F. J. Cleton, pp. 397–412. M. Nijhoff Publishers, The Hague, The Netherlands.
33. Savlov, E. D., Knight, E., MacIntyre, J. M., and Wolter, J. (1981): Comparison of adriamycin with cycloleucine in the treatment of sarcomas. *Cancer Treat. Rep. (in press)*.
34. Sordillo, P., Magill, G. B., Howard, J., and Golbey, R. B. (1978): Adjuvant chemotherapy of adult soft part sarcomas with "ALOMAD." *Proc. Am. Soc. Clin. Oncol.*, 19:353.
35. Stewart, D. J., Benjamin, R. S., Baker, L., Yap, B. S., and Bodey, G. P. (1980): New drugs for the treatment of soft tissue sarcoma. In: *International Course on Recent Advances in the Treatment of Ovarian and Testicular Cancer and of Soft Tissue and Bone Sarcoma*, edited by A. T. Van Oosterom, F. M. Muggia, and F. J. Cleton, pp. 453–479. M. Nijhoff Publishers, The Hague, The Netherlands.
36. Subramanian, S., and Wiltshaw, E. (1978): Chemotherapy of sarcoma. *Lancet*, 1:686–693.
37. Wiltshaw, E., Harmer, C., and McKinna, A. (1980): Soft tissue sarcoma: Treatment of advanced disease in the Royal Marsden Hospital. In: *International Course on Recent Advances in the*

Treatment of Ovarian and Testicular Cancer and of Soft Tissue and Bone Sarcomas, edited by A. T. Van Oosterom, F. M. Muggia, and F. J. Cleton, pp. 413–423. M. Nijhoff Publishers, The Hague, The Netherlands.

38. Yap, B. S., Baker, L. H., Sinkovics, J. G., and Rivkin, S. (1980): Cyclophosphamide, vincristine, adriamycin, and DTIC (CYVADIC) combination chemotherapy for the treatment of advanced sarcomas. *Cancer Treat. Rep.*, 64:93–98.
39. Yap, B. S., Sinkovics, J. G., Benjamin, R. S., and Bodey, G. P. (1979): Survival and relapse patterns of complete responders in adults with advanced soft tissue sarcomas (STS). *Proc. Am. Soc. Clin. Oncol.*, 20:352.

New Approaches in Cancer Therapy,
edited by H. Cortés Funes and M. Rozencweig.
Raven Press, New York © 1982.

Combination Chemotherapy for Advanced Head and Neck Tumors with Two Different Regimens

G. Perez Manga, P. Madrigal Alonso, and M. Fernandez Vega

Hospital Oncológico Provincial, Madrid, Spain

There is still a great number of patients with head and neck cancers that can be treated with chemotherapy, after the failure of surgery and/or radiotherapy. Several drugs, such as methotrexate, hydroxyurea, vinblastine, bleomycin, cisplatin, adriamycin, etc., have shown their effectiveness in the treatment of these tumors (18). At the present time, the most useful agent is methotrexate given as intermittent weekly or biweekly injections (5).

Vincristine is of little use as single agent for head and neck tumors (2). When associated with methotrexate, it seems to potentiate the efficacy of the antimetabolite (4). When both drugs are combined, a 53% regression rate may be obtained (14). Bleomycin has been extensively studied in squamous cell carcinoma of the head and neck, although its efficacy is clearly inferior to methotrexate as single agent. The overall response rate is 38% (18). Adriamycin has produced regressions in 23% of the patients treated (18). The association of adriamycin and bleomycin achieved 50% of objective responses in one series (3).

The sensitivity of this type of tumor to chemotherapy seems to have been clearly demonstrated; at present there are several regimens that show a response rate superior to 50% (14–16). Unfortunately, the duration of response and the survival increase obtained is still disappointing when patients in advanced stages are treated.

The study described herein was designed in 1975 in an attempt to prolong the survival rate in relapsing patients by using two different non-cross-resistant combination chemotherapy regimens with proven efficacy.

MATERIAL AND METHODS

Ninety-four patients with clinically advanced stage 3 and 4 histologically confirmed squamous cell carcinoma of the head and neck have been eligible for this study since 1975. To be eligible, patients must have measurable lesions, performance status >40%, (Karnofsky scale), normal renal function (serum creatinine <1.7 mg%), adequate pulmonary function (vital capacity >75% predicted normal level), adequate bone marrow reserve (white blood cells >4,000/mm³ and platelet count

>100,000/mm^3), and normal electrocardiogram. Prior to initiation of therapy, every patient underwent complete work-up including physical examination to assess extent of disease.

Patients with prior chemotherapy were considered ineligible for the study. All patients had been previously treated with surgery and/or radiation therapy to primary tumor and regional lymph nodes. Age ranged from 17 to 70 years with a median of 56. There were 85 males and 9 females. The primary tumor localization, site of relapse, prior therapy, and cell differentiation in these patients are described in Table 1.

Forty-five patients showed only one tumor localization. From these, 4 were distant metastases, 26 were regional lymph node relapses, and 15 had local tumor relapse as the only manifestation of the disease. The rest of the patients had multiple tumor localizations, mainly regional lymph nodes plus local relapse or distant metastases. Distant metastases were present mainly in the lung. This was seen in 21 patients; 2 other patients had metastatic disease in bones and liver. Only 2 patients with metastases had a high degree of tumor cell differentiation. The remaining patients had tumors with moderate or poor differentiation.

There were no statistical differences between the treatment groups as to sex, localization of the primary or relapsed tumor, cell differentiation, previous treatment, performance status, and disease-free interval.

TABLE 1. *Patient characteristics*

	Regimen A	Regimen B	Regimens A and B
Number	56	38	94
Sex			
Female	4	5	9
Male	52	33	85
Age			
Median	58	54	56
Range	40–70	17–70	17–70
Primary localization			
Laryngopharynx	35	24	59 (63%)
Tongue	10	5	15 (16%)
Lips	7	4	11 (12%)
Nasopharynx	4	5	9 (9%)
Site of relapse			
Primary	39	42	81 (69%)
Nodes	48	46	94 (80%)
Lung, bone, or liver	12	11	23 (23%)
Prior therapy			
Surgery	52	39	91 (89%)
Radiotherapy	53	43	96 (94%)
Histological differentiation			
Well	16	16	32 (34%)
Moderate	32	14	46 (49%)
Poor	8	8	16 (17%)

Patients were randomized to receive one of two different regimens. Patients on regimen A received a combination of methotrexate, 30 mg/m^2 i.v., on days 1, 8, and 15, and vincristine, 1 mg/m^2, the same days repeated at 2-week intervals. In regimen B, patients were treated with a combination of bleomycin, 10 mg/m^2 i.v., days 1 and 8, and adriamycin, 40 mg/m^2 i.v., day 1, both repeated every 3 weeks. There were 56 patients treated with regimen A and 38 with regimen B. Relapsed or initially nonresponding patients were crossed over to the other regimen and a second evaluation of response was done.

Dosages of adriamycin and methotrexate were adjusted according to hematologic toxicity and discontinued or delayed when white blood cells were below 1,500/mm^3 and/or platelets were below 100,000/mm^3. In the presence of persisting neurological toxicity, vincristine was discontinued until recovery. The dose of methotrexate and bleomycin was reduced to 50% if severe mucositis was detected. Adriamycin and bleomycin were given at the maximum dosages of 450 mg/m^2 and 300 units/m^2, respectively.

All patients were evaluated for tumor responses at 3- to 4-week intervals. Complete response (CR) was the total disappearance of all measurable disease. A partial response (PR) was more than 50% reduction in the sum of the products of two diameters of measurable lesions. Minor response (MR) was a 25 to 50% reduction in the sum of two diameters of measurable lesions. A minimal duration of response required 4 weeks to be accepted as tumor response. Stable disease (SD) was one in which the tumor shrank by 25% or remained unchanged during therapy. Progressive disease (PD) was defined as any objective increase of size of tumor at any time. Survival duration was calculated from the date of initial chemotherapy.

RESULTS

The overall response rate was 37.5% and 36.8%, respectively, with regimen A and B (Table 2). There were an additional 20% and 22% of MR or stabilizations in each of the group. Four patients from group A (7%) and 1 patient from group B (3%) achieved CR, and 17 and 13, respectively, achieved PR, with no statistical difference between the two groups. There was a statistically significant difference in response rate in relation to prior chemotherapy ($p < 0.05$). Patients with prior chemotherapy responded better to regimen A than to regimen B.

Responses were generally noted within 4 weeks although some responses continued to improve up to 3 months.

Table 3 gives the response rate according to initial performance status, site of primary disease, and cell differentiation. There are no apparent differences in response rate between fully ambulatory and partially ambulatory patients. There are also no differences according to the original primary site.

The median duration of remission was 4.9 months for the regimen A group and 5.1 for the regimen B group ($p > 0.3$).

The median survival for the patients who responded to regimen A was 11.2 months and 7.4 for those who failed to respond ($p > 0.3$). The responders to

TABLE 2. *Responses*

	Regimen A	Regimen B
No prior chemotherapy		
CR	4/56 (7%)	1/38 (3%)
PR	17/56 (30%)	13/38 (34%)
CR + PR	21/56 (37%)	14/38 (37%)
Cross-over		
CR + PR	2/10 (20%)	1/13 (7%)

TABLE 3. *Objective responses by characteristics*

	Group A	Group B
By cell differentiation		
Well	3/16 (19%)	4/16 (25%)
Moderate	15/32 (47%)	11/14 (79%)
Poor	5/8	4/8
By primary site		
Laryngopharynx	14/35 (40%)	10/34 (29%)
Tongue	3/10 (30%)	1/5
Lips	2/7	1/4
Nasopharynx	2/4	2/5
By prior therapy		
Radiotherapy	18/53 (34%)	16/43 (37%)
No radiotherapy	2/3	2/5
By performance status		
Fully ambulatory	16/43 (37%)	9/25 (36%)
Partially ambulatory	4/11 (36%)	4/13 (31%)

regimen B had a median survival of 8.2 months compared to 3 months in nonresponders (Figs. 1 and 2).

All patients who achieved a CR are still alive and free of disease 4 years later. In 3 of the patients previously treated with chemotherapy who responded, the duration of the remission was 2, 3, and 2 months; survival from the beginning of the second chemotherapy treatment was 3, 4, and 4 months, respectively.

Toxicity with both regimens was generally mild (Table 4). White blood cells were below 3,000 in 30% of the patients in group A and 34% in group B; platelets were below 10,000 in 6% of the patients in group A and 11% in group B. Alopecia was more frequent in regimen B (66%) than A (20%) and patients also had more vomiting with regimen B (45% versus 30%). Neurotoxicity due to vincristine occurred in 39% of the patients treated with regimen A. Most patients were able to tolerate full doses of drugs for the first 4 months. Some dose reduction was required because of myelosuppression.

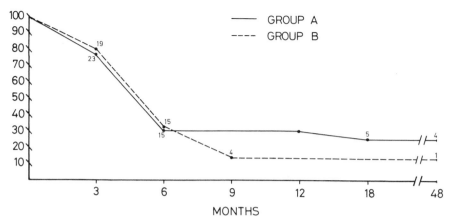

FIG. 1. Actuarial relapse.

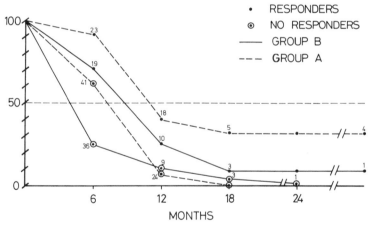

FIG. 2. Actuarial survival.

DISCUSSION

Chemotherapy plays an important role in the treatment of head and neck tumors. This role is not only for palliation but, possibly, also for cure in association with surgery and/or radiation therapy. In this study we tried to determine if patients responding to chemotherapy had an increase in survival using one of two different combination chemotherapy regimens without cross-resistance. At the same time, we tried to analyze the different prognostic factors that may influence response to chemotherapy. Patients who responded to chemotherapy in both arms of the study have better survival compared to nonresponders. However, this difference was not statistically significant ($p > 0.3$).

TABLE 4. *Toxicity*

	Group A	Group B
White blood cells <3,000	17/56 (30%)	13/38 (34%)
Platelets <100,000	3/56 (5%)	4/38 (11%)
Alopecia	11/56 (20%)	25/38 (66%)
Mucositis	12/56 (21%)	8/38 (21%)
Vomiting	17/56 (30%)	17/38 (45%)
Neurotoxicity	22/56 (39%)	0/38 (0%)
Heart	0/56 (0%)	3/38 (8%)
Lung fibrosis	0/56 (0%)	2/38 (5%)
Fever	0/56 (0%)	16/38 (42%)

Survival seems to be clearly increased in those patients with CR of the tumors after treatment. Patients who failed first-line regimen and were crossed over rarely responded to the other combination therapy (only 3 out of 23). There was no increase in survival. Results were better in patients without previous radiotherapy and in those who had undergone surgery, but differences were not statistically significant, probably due to the small number of patients not treated with surgery or who had received radiotherapy. Patients without prior chemotherapy responded better to treatment. The difference was statistically significant ($p < 0.05$).

Contrary to other published results (1,16), in our study, patients with poorly differentiated tumors responded significantly better to the chemotherapy than patients with moderately and well-differentiated ones ($p < 0.05$ and $p < 0.02$, respectively), including better response to the bleomycin combination, which, in accordance with other authors, should be more active in well-differentiated tumors (7).

The site of the primary tumors has been considered an initial prognostic factor by a number of authors (1,18); however, the results achieved for the different tumor sites were not significantly different in our study. The real importance of this factor is probably more complex, since it frequently is indirectly determined by the modality of local treatments and, more or less frequently by the degree of tumor differentiation. This relationship can explain why the best response rate corresponded in our trial to tumors of the cavum, usually poorly differentiated. Tumors with a high degree of differentiation, all of them previously treated with surgery and radiotherapy, had the worst results.

The overall response rate of the chemotherapy regimens used in our study is low compared with the results reported by Nervi et al. (14) and Cortes et al. (3) using the same combinations. The number of patients included in our series can, in our opinion, justify these differences. The response rate to the regimen of adriamycin and bleomycin is superior to that achieved with the same drugs used as single agents (5,18). However, no synergism between these two drugs seems to exist when they are combined.

Our results with regimen A (vincristine and methotrexate) were inferior to those reported with methotrexate alone (8,9,13,18). The overall remission rate of our protocol is comparable to that obtained with COMB and BACOM (12), BCAM (19) and BCOAML (10),[1] whereas it is superior to the results of bleomycin and vincristine in combination (11). Results reported by several investigators with a variety of combinations (6,15,17) are better when compared with the results of our regimens. However, the duration of responses was similar. From these data, we can conclude that our regimens may be recommended as effective and safe outpatient treatment of epidermoid carcinomas of the head and neck.

Histological degree and previous treatments are the two most important prognostic factors for the response to chemotherapy in our series. The prognostic values of other factors, such as performance status, sex, site of primary location or relapse, etc., still need to be confirmed.

Only CR seems to prolong the survival of the patients. Further efforts must be made to develop new regimens more effective than single agent methotrexate. Another approach should be to use chemotherapy earlier in the initial treatment of these patients, as part of a well-planned multidisciplinary approach.

REFERENCES

1. Bertino, J. R., Boston, B., and Capizzi, R. L. (1975): The role of chemotherapy in the management of cancer of head and neck: A review. *Cancer*, 36:752.
2. Carter, S. K., Bakowski, M. T., and Hellmann, K. (1977): *Chemotherapy of Cancer*, pp. 205–209. John Wiley & Sons, New York.
3. Cortes, E. P., Shedd, D., and Albert, D. J. (1972): Adriamycin and bleomycin in advanced cancer. *Proc. Am. Assoc. Cancer Res.*, 13:86.
4. Goldman, I. D. (1975): Membrane transport of methotrexate (NSC-740) and other folate compounds: Relevance to rescue protocols. *Cancer Chemother. Rep.*, 6:63–72.
5. Goldsmith, M. A., and Carter, S. K. (1975): The integration of chemotherapy into combined modality approach to cancer therapy. *Cancer Treat. Rev.*, 2:137–158.
6. Hanham, I. W. F., New, K. A., and Westburg, G. (1971): Seventy-five cases of solid tumors treated by a modified quadruple chemotherapy regimen. *Br. J. Cancer*, 25:462–478.
7. Ichikawa, T. (1968): Bleomycin: A new tumor antibiotic (as a specific agent against squamous cell carcinoma). *J. Jap. Med. Assoc.*, 61:478.
8. Lane, M., Moore, J. E., and Levin, H. (1968): Methotrexate therapy for squamous cell carcinoma of the head and neck. *JAMA*, 204:561–564.
9. Leone, L. A., Albalba, M. M., and Rege, V. B. (1968): Treatment of carcinoma of the head and neck with intravenous methotrexate. *Cancer*, 21:828–837.
10. Lester, E. P., Kinnealey, A., and Matz, G. J. (1979): Sequential combination chemotherapy for advanced squamous cell carcinoma of the head and neck. *Laryngoscope*, 89:1,921–1,929.
11. Livingston, R. B., Bodey, G., Gottlieb, J., and Frey, E. (1975): Kinetic scheduling of vincristine and other malignant tumors. *Cancer Chemother. Rep.*, 57:219–224.
12. Livingston, R. B., Einhorn, L. H., Burgess, M. A., and Gottlieb, J. A. (1976): Sequential combination chemotherapy for advanced, recurrent squamous carcinoma of the head and neck. *Cancer Treat. Rep.*, 1:103–105.

---

[1]COMB: cyclophosphamide, vincristine, methotrexate, and bleomycin. BACOM: bleomycin, adriamycin, cyclophosphamide, vincristine, and methotrexate. BCAM: bleomycin, cyclophosphamide, adriamycin, and methotrexate. BCOAML: bleomycin, cyclophosphamide, vincristine, adriamycin, methotrexate, and leucovorin.

13. Mosher, M. B., Deconti, R. C., and Bertino, J. R. (1972): Bleomycin therapy in advanced Hodgkin's disease and epidermoid cancer. *Cancer*, 30:56–60.
14. Nervi, C., Casale, C., and Cortese, M. (1969): Combination of low doses of vincristine with high doses of methotrexate in the therapy of solid tumors. *Tumori*, 55:103–111.
15. Pouillart, P., and Mathe, G. (1976): Bleomycin in rational combinations of chemotherapy. *GANN Monograph on Cancer Research. N°19. Fundamental and Clinical Studies of Bleomycin*, pp. 279–283. University of Tokyo Press, Tokyo.
16. Price, L. A., and Hill, B. T. (1977): A kinetically based logical approach to the chemotherapy of head and neck cancer. *Clin. Otorrinol.*, 2:339–354.
17. Price, L. A., Hill, B. T., Calvert, A. H., Dalley, M., Levene, A., Busby, E. R., Schachter, M., and Shaw, H. J. (1978): Improved results in combination chemotherapy of head and neck cancer using a kinetically based approach: A randomized study with and without adriamycin. *Oncology*, 35:26–28.
18. Taylor, S. G. (1977): Head and neck cancer. In: *Manual for Staging of Cancer*, pp. 237–256. American Joint Committee for stating and end results reporting, Chicago, Illinois.
19. Wittes, R. E., Spiro, R. H., Shah, J., Gerold, F. P., Koven, B., and Strong, E. W. (1977): Chemotherapy of head and neck cancer: Combination treatment with cyclophosphamide, adriamycin, methotrexate and bleomycin. *Med. Pediatr. Oncol.*, 3:301–309.

New Approaches in Cancer Therapy,
edited by H. Cortés Funes and M. Rozencweig.
Raven Press, New York © 1982.

Cisplatin, Methotrexate, Bleomycin, and Vincristine: An Effective Combination Chemotherapy Regimen in Squamous Cell Carcinoma of the Head and Neck

*P. Dodion, **U. Bruntsch, **W. Gallmeier, †M. Clavel,
†B. Gignoux, ‡F. Cavalli, §H. Cortés Funes, §§J. Wildiers,
#A. Kirkpatrick, #O. Dalesio, and *M. Rozencweig for the
EORTC Head and Neck Cooperative Group

*Institut Jules Bordet, Brussels, Belgium; **5. Medizinische Klinik, Nurnberg, West
Germany; †Centre Léon Bérard, Lyon, France; ‡Ospedale San Giovanni, Bellinzona,
Switzerland; §Hospital "1° Octubre," Madrid, Spain; §§Akademisch Ziekenhuis St
Rafael, Leuven, Belgium; and #EORTC/Data Center, Brussels, Belgium

The management of head and neck cancer is a challenging problem for medical oncologists. This disease occurs principally among elderly patients and is relatively infrequent, i.e., 5% of all malignancies in the United States. The use of chemotherapy is generally restricted to tumors beyond the control of surgery and radiotherapy. At this stage of the disease, rapidly declining performance status and lack of clearly evaluable lesions often hamper the administration of cytotoxic agents. Moreover, little effect of systemic treatment can be expected in diseases relapsing in previously operated and irradiated areas.

Despite these unfavorable characteristics, a number of active compounds have been identified, resulting in the recently expanding investigation of various combination chemotherapy regimens (14). High response rates reported in nonrandomized trials with these newly developed regimens could be biased by variations in patient selection, response criteria, and method of data reporting. Few studies have randomly compared single-agent and combination chemotherapy programs. Results of these studies have been mostly published in an abstract form providing insufficient information for critical analyses. Some studies have accrued too small numbers of patients to detect significant differences. Others have investigated combinations including agents of uncertain activity. The reference arm has been either methotrexate or cisplatin. A single trial has shown a superiority of the combination.

Stimulating results were reported by Kaplan et al. (9) with a combination of cisplatin, methotrexate, and bleomycin, given on an outpatient basis. Among 46 evaluable patients, 8 achieved complete remission (CR) and 21 partial remission

(PR), for an overall response rate of 62%. Toxicity was relatively mild in this trial. This combination was subsequently compared to methotrexate 40 mg/m² i.v. weekly in a randomized trial conducted by ECOG (8). Ninety-six percent of the of the patients had received prior radiotherapy. Interim results with 61 evaluable patients in each treatment arm indicated a CR and PR rate of 18 and 28%, respectively, for the combination versus 7 and 19% for methotrexate. Although this difference was significant, median time-to-progression in responding patients and survival were similar in either treatment arm.

The Eastern Cooperative Oncology Group (ECOG) had previously investigated the efficacy of methotrexate 40 mg/m² i.v. weekly versus biweekly methotrexate 240 mg/m² i.v. followed by leucovorin rescue versus a combination of methotrexate, leucovorin, cyclophosphamide, and cytosine arabinoside (6). Among 191 evaluable patients, the overall response rate was 24% with no significant difference between the three treatment options. The median duration of all responses approximated 50 days.

The same reference arm of weekly methotrexate was tested versus a combination of cisplatin, vincristine, and bleomycin (1). A total of 40 patients were evaluated. These treatments achieved similar response rates (40 versus 45%), response duration, and overall survival.

In an ongoing trial of the Southeastern Cancer Study Group, weekly methotrexate is being compared to a combination of cisplatin, vinblastine, and bleomycin. No results are available as yet.

Methotrexate 15 mg/m² i.m. 3 times daily every 3 weeks was compared to a regimen consisting of methotrexate, bleomycin, and semustine (methylCCNU) (12). A total of 196 fully and partially evaluable patients were entered. The overall complete plus partial response rate was 33% with methotrexate and 26% with the combination. Median survival for all patients was 29 and 14 weeks, respectively.

Davis and Kessler randomly allocated 57 patients to receive cisplatin alone or in combination with methotrexate and bleomycin (5). All patients had received prior radiotherapy. Overall response rates were 13 and 11%, respectively.

Finally, in an ongoing trial of the Northern California Oncology Group, cisplatin alone is being compared to a regimen consisting of cisplatin, methotrexate, and leucovorin rescue. Interim data were presented with a total of 37 patients (7). Results were coded and showed response rates of 13 versus 31% and median survival times of 179 versus 204 days. None of these differences were statistically significant.

In 1979, the EORTC Head and Neck Cooperative Group initiated a study of the combination of cisplatin, methotrexate, and bleomycin as designed by Kaplan et al. (9), plus vincristine (CABO). Considering all the trials that were ongoing elsewhere at that time, a nonrandomized design was chosen. This chapter reports an interim analysis of this study.

MATERIAL AND METHODS

Patients with inoperable, recurrent, and/or metastatic squamous cell carcinoma of the head and neck were eligible for the trial. Other eligibility criteria included the presence of measurable lesions, no prior treatment with any of the drugs used in this study, a performance status on the Karnofsky scale of 50 or more, age ≤ 75 years, white blood cell count (WBC) ≥ 4,000/mm³, platelet counts ≥ 100,000/mm³, and creatinine and bilirubin serum levels < 1.5 mg%. Patients with marked senility, uncontrolled infections, or expected difficulties in the follow-up were excluded from the trial. Informed consent was obtained from each patient according to local institutional policies.

The treatment regimen consisted of methotrexate 40 mg/m² i.v. or i.m. days 1 and 15, bleomycin 10 mg i.v. or i.m. days 1, 8, and 15, vincristine 2 mg i.v. on days 1, 8, and 15, and cisplatin 50 mg/m² i.v. on day 4. Cisplatin was given 30 min after the beginning of an i.v. infusion of dextrose 5% in ½ normal saline + 10 mEq KCl/liter at a rate of 1 liter/hr for 2 hr. Forced diuresis was obtained with furosemide and mannitol. Cycles were repeated every 3 weeks. Vincristine was withdrawn after 6 doses and bleomycin after a cumulative dose of 400 mg. This regimen was suitable for outpatient treatments.

An adequate trial required at least two courses of therapy. CR was defined as a complete disappearance of all clinically detectable disease for at least 4 weeks. PR was defined as a greater than 50% decrease in the sum of the products of the largest perpendicular diameters of malignant lesions for at least 4 weeks. An increase of 25% in the sum of the products of the largest diameters of malignant lesions or the appearance of any new lesion was considered as a progression. Patients who failed to meet the criteria of CR, PR, or progression were considered as having stable disease.

A Student's *t* test was used for statistical analyses.

RESULTS

At the time of this analysis, 127 patients were entered in the study by 13 institutions. Twenty-nine were ineligible because of nonevaluable lesions (20), prior chemotherapy with one of the drugs included in this regimen (7), renal insufficiency prior to therapy (1), and performance status below 50 (1). No information was available for 1 entered patient. Of the 97 eligible patients, 55 were evaluable for response and toxicity, 26 were not yet evaluated, 11 received less than two courses of therapy, and 5 were treated with major protocol violations.

Among evaluable patients, median age was 54 with a range of 35 to 74 years; median performance status on the Karnofsky scale was 80 with a range of 50 to 100 (Table 1). All but 3 were men. About ½ of the patients had been treated with surgery (27), radiotherapy (26), and/or chemotherapy (5), whereas 23 patients had not received any prior therapy. Thirty-eight patients had locoregional disease and 17 had distant metastases. The most frequent primary sites were the larynx (19), the oropharynx (7), and the hypopharynx (7). The median number of courses was three with a range of 2 to 11.

Eight patients achieved CR and 28 achieved PR for an overall response rate of 65.5% (Table 2). Twelve patients had stable disease and 7 had progression after

TABLE 1. *Pretreatment characteristics of the 55 evaluable patients*

Median age (range)	54 (35–74)
Median Karnofsky index (range)	80 (50–100)
Men/women	52/3
No prior therapy	23
Prior surgery	27
Prior radiotherapy	26
Prior chemotherapy	5
Locoregional/distant metastases	38/17

TABLE 2. *Response to therapy*

	No. of patients	Response rate (%)
Complete response	8	14.5
Partial response	28	51
No change	12	
Progression	7	
	55	

TABLE 3. *Time-to-response and response duration*

		Median no. of weeks (range)		
Best response	No. of patients	Time to PR	Time to CR	Duration of best response
Partial	28	5 (3–10)		10+ (6+ – 39)
Complete	8	3 (1–4)	7 (1–12)	9+ (6+ – 23+)

two courses. Time-to-response was generally short, with a median time-to-PR and -to-CR of 5 and 7 weeks, respectively (Table 3). All patients who achieved CR had tumor shrinkage by at least 50% after 4 weeks of therapy. Thirty-seven % of patients who achieved PR did so within one course of therapy, 81.5% within two courses, 96.3% within three courses, and all within four courses. Corresponding figures for CR were 37%, 50%, 94.3%, and 100%, respectively. The median duration of PR was 10+ weeks (range, 6+ to 39) and that of CR was 9+ weeks (range, 6+ to 23+). Response duration was difficult to interpret in this trial since 15 patients received other treatment modalities while responding to chemotherapy. Among the 21 remaining responders, 8 were still responding.

Response rate was significantly higher in patients with a performance status of 90 or 100 relative to those with a lower performance status ($p = 0.03$) (Table 4).

TABLE 4. *Response by pretreatment characteristics*

Characteristic	No. of patients	Overall response rate (%)
Performance status		
≤80	31	52
90–100	24	79
Prior radiotherapy		
yes	26	54
no	29	76
Prior surgery		
yes	27	59
no	28	71
Prior chemotherapy		
yes	5	40
no	50	68

TABLE 5. *Response by extent of disease and prior radiotherapy*

	No. of patients			Overall response rate (%)
	Total	CR	PR	
Locoregional, no prior RT	22	5	11	73
All others	33	3	17	60
Locoregional, prior RT	16	2	5	44
Distant metastases	17	1	12	76

Patients with prior or no prior radiotherapy showed a response rate of 54 versus 76%. This difference approached statistical significance ($p = 0.076$). Results in patients with locoregional disease and no prior radiotherapy were similar to those in patients with distant metastases, whereas data were distinctly less favorable in patients with locoregional disease and prior radiation therapy (Table 5). This observation further pointed to the chemoresistance of irradiated lesions. Response rate was diminished in patients who had prior surgery, but most of these had also prior radiotherapy (data not shown). Prior chemotherapy also seemed to adversely affect response rate. Age, extent of disease, and primary site did not appear to be of major prognostic significance.

Myelosuppression was evaluable in 53 patients (Table 6). Thirty percent of the patients had no leukopenia, 51% experienced mild to moderate leukopenia with WBC remaining above 2,000/mm^3, and 19% had severe leukopenia. There were 9 episodes of infection; only 2 were related to leukopenia, and 1 of these was life-threatening. Thrombocytopenia was minimal. There was no treatment-related hemorrhage. There was a trend suggesting more severe myelosuppression in previously irradiated patients as compared to those with no prior radiotherapy.

TABLE 6. *Drug-induced myelosuppression in 53 evaluable patients*

Nadir	No. of patients (%)
WBC × 10³/mm³	
≥4.0	16 (30)
3.0–3.9	10 (19)
2.0–2.9	17 (32)
1.0–1.9	7 (13)
<1.0	3 (6)
Platelets × 10³/mm³	
≥100	43 (81)
50–99	8 (15)
<50	2 (4)

TABLE 7. *Nonhematological toxic effects*

Toxic effect	No. of toxic patients (%)	Mild to moderate	Severe to life-threatening
Nausea/vomiting	49 (89)	42	7
Alopecia	31 (56)	24	7
Neurological	31 (56)	25	6
Stomatitis	15 (27)	12	3
Fever/chills	13 (24)	10	3
Respiratory	10 (18)	9	1
Infection	9 (16)	6	3
Skin	6 (11)	3	3
Renal	5 (9)	5	0
Bleeding	4 (7)	4	0
Hepatic	2 (4)	2	0

Nonhematological toxic effects (Table 7) included primarily nausea and vomiting, which were experienced by 89% of the patients and were severe in 15% of these. Alopecia and neurotoxicity, consisting mainly of paresthesia, were encountered in 56% of the patients. Stomatitis occurred in 27% of the patients, but was generally mild or moderate. Fever and chills were seen in 24% of the patients, generally after bleomycin injection. Pulmonary toxicity was found in 10 patients who had bibasilar rales but no histologically proven fibrosis. Skin toxicity was seen in 6 patients. Mild and reversible renal impairment occurred in 5 patients, but creatinine levels never exceeded 3.5 mg% and complete recovery was obtained within 1 to 5 weeks. Hepatic toxicity, consisting of slight and reversible alterations of transaminases, was noted in 2 patients.

DISCUSSION

In squamous cell cancer of the head and neck, single-agent chemotherapy may achieve response rates of 20 to 30%, with rare CR (14). With current combination chemotherapy programs, response rates of 50% are commonly obtained, especially in single institutional studies. In this trial, we investigated the antitumor activity of a combination of cisplatin, methotrexate, bleomycin, and vincristine. The overall response rate of 66% that was obtained seemed of particular interest, considering the cooperative nature of the trial.

The contribution of vincristine to CABO is disputable. The apparent superiority of this four-drug combination over the same combination without vincristine, based on ECOG results (8), might be largely accounted for by differences in data analysis and selection of patients with particular respect to prior radiotherapy. These factors could also explain the markedly less impressive findings of King et al. (11) with a combination of the four drugs used in our study. In this case, however, lower response rate could also result from lower dosage of chemotherapy.

Although response rates have increased with polychemotherapy, duration of response remains, generally, disappointingly low (Table 8). In the randomized trial conducted by ECOG, there was no advantage of the combination of methotrexate, cisplatin, and bleomycin over methotrexate alone in terms of response duration (8). It is still premature to assess this variable in our trial; moreover, figures might be artificially lowered by the exclusion from this analysis of favorable patients who received additional treatment while responding to chemotherapy.

The toxicity of CABO may be considered as generally acceptable with the exception of cisplatin-induced gastrointestinal intolerance. Nausea and vomiting were frequent and contributed sometimes to treatment refusal. Neurotoxicity was mild and did not appear to be more serious than that seen with cisplatin or vincristine alone.

Of particular interest, renal toxicity was low despite the inclusion of methotrexate and cisplatin in the regimen. This observation largely confirms data previously reported by Kaplan et al. (9).

Thus, our chemotherapy regimen appears to be quite effective in inducing rapid tumor regression with acceptable toxicity. This trial is closed for patient accrual and, although definite conclusions must still await a final analysis, these interim results have served as a basis to design subsequent generation studies within EORTC.

From initial data with CABO and experience with other regimens of similar efficacy, it would appear that long-lasting remissions are unlikely to occur with our four-drug combination. In patients no longer suitable for surgery or radiotherapy, our therapeutic strategy is currently aimed at defining a treatment program that may achieve high response rates with less toxicity and discomfort. Possibly non-cross-resistant combinations are also investigated. In addition, the potential of aggressive induction chemotherapy prior to surgery and radiotherapy is evaluated.

Our first-line chemotherapy trial is studying the contribution of cisplatin to our four-drug regimen using a randomized design (CABO versus ABO): cisplatin is the drug causing the most important toxic effects in the CABO regimen and, in addition, a combination of low-dose vincristine, bleomycin, and methotrexate was found by Molinari et al. (13) to yield an overall response rate of 62% with relatively mild toxic effects. In the current protocol, patients receive three courses of either com-

TABLE 8. *Rate and duration of response to chemotherapy*

Ref.	Treatment[a]	Overall response rate (%)	Median duration of response (months)
Brown (3)	DDP-BLM-VCR	60	4.0
Caradonna (4)	DDP-BLM-MTX	74	4.0
King (11)	DDP-BLM-MTX-VCR	24	6.0
Kaplan (10)	DDP-BLM-MTX-MMC	62	4.0
Molinari (13)	BLM-MTX-VCR	62	4.0
Ratkin (15)	BLM-MTX-VCR	52	4.7
Woods (17)	BLM-MTX-VCR	24	4.5
Wittes (16)	BLM-MTX-CTX-ADM	35	3.0

[a]DDP: cisplatin; BLM: bleomycin; VCR: vincristine; MTX: methotrexate; MMC: mitomycin-C; CTX: cyclophosphamide; ADM: adriamycin.

bination and are then maintained on weekly methotrexate alone, since best response was obtained within three courses of therapy in about 90% of the patients in our previous CABO trial.

Two second-line chemotherapy trials have also been designed. Patients with prior treatment with one of the drugs used in these studies are ineligible. One protocol is testing a regimen consisting of hydroxyurea, mitomycin C, and 5-fluorouracil which all have been reported in the older literature to have single-agent activity in head and neck cancer (14). The other protocol investigates the value of cisplatin and 5-fluorouracil in combination, in light of excellent results reported by Al-Sarraf et al. in previously untreated patients (2).

Finally, a nonrandomized pilot trial has been designed for patients with T3-T4 and/or N3 squamous cell carcinoma of the head and neck suitable for definitive local therapy. All patients receive initially two to three courses of our CABO regimen. Patients are then allocated to one of two treatment options according to the site of origin of the primary and the nodal status.

Patients with tumors of the buccal mucosa, osseous palate, superior gingiva, oropharynx, or rhinopharynx with N0, N1, or N2 lymph node status and patients with any primary site with N3 lymph node status are irradiated with 7,000 rad in a field defined according to prechemotherapy findings, unless the disease has progressed since. Residual disease is removed surgically. A radical neck node dissection is performed for residual lymph nodes.

Patients with tumors of the tongue, floor of the mouth, inferior gingiva, hypopharynx, or larynx with N0, N1, or N2 lymph node status undergo surgery, the extent of which is defined prior to chemotherapy, unless progression has occurred since. Patients with incompletely resected tumors and/or pathologically involved regional lymph nodes at operation receive subsequently radiotherapy with 5,000 rad to a field delineated in accordance to the extent of disease prior to chemotherapy plus a boost of 1,000 to 1,500 rad to areas of incompletely resected tumor deposits and/or cervical lymph nodes with capsular rupture.

The Southwest Oncology Group (SWOG) has recently activated a randomized trial testing the value of preoperative chemotherapy in stage III or IV squamous cell carcinoma of the oral cavity, oropharynx, hypopharynx, or larynx. The chemotherapy program is based on the combination developed by King et al. (11) with further dosage reduction. Results of these SWOG and EORTC trials are awaited with great expectations.

ACKNOWLEDGMENTS

This study was supported in part by contract NIH N01/CM53840 from the National Cancer Institute (Bethesda, Maryland) and by grant 3.4535.79 from the "Fonds de la Recherche Scientifique Médicale" (Brussels, Belgium).

The authors acknowledge the secretarial assistance of Mrs. Geneviève Decoster.

REFERENCES

1. Al-Sarraf, M. (1980): The clinical value of cis-platinum, oncovin, and bleomycin (COB) combination vs standard single agent in advanced epidermoid cancer of the head and neck. *Proceedings of the NCI International Head and Neck Oncology Research Conference*, Abstract 2-13.
2. Al-Sarraf, M., Drelichman, A., Peppard, S., Hoschner, J., Kinzie, J., Loh, J., and Weaver, A. (1981): Adjuvant cis-platinum and 5-fluorouracil 96-hour infusion in previously untreated epidermoid cancers of the head and neck. *Proc. Am. Assoc. Cancer Res. and ASCO*, 22:428.
3. Brown, A. W., Blom, J., Butler, W. M., Garcia-Guerrero, G., Richardson, M. F., and Henderson, R. L. (1980): Combination chemotherapy with vinblastine, bleomycin, and cis-diamminedichloroplatinum (II) in squamous cell carcinoma of the head and neck. *Cancer*, 45:2,830–2,835.
4. Caradonna, R., Paladine, W., Ruckdeschel, J. C., Goldstein, J. C., Olson, J. E., Jaski, J. W., Silvers, S. A., Hillinger, S., and Horton, J. (1979): Methotrexate, bleomycin, and high-dose cis-dichlorodiammineplatinum (II) in the treatment of advanced epidermoid carcinoma of the head and neck. *Cancer Treat. Rep.*, 63:489–491.
5. Davis, S., and Kessler, W. (1979): Randomized comparison of cis-diamminedichloroplatinum versus cis-diamminedichloroplatinum, methotrexate, and bleomycin in recurrent squamous cell carcinoma of the head and neck. *Cancer Chemother. Pharmacol.*, 3:57–59.
6. DeConti, R. C. for the Eastern Cooperative Oncology Group (1976): Phase III comparison of methotrexate with leucovorin vs methotrexate alone vs a combination of methotrexate plus leucovorin, cyclophosphamide, and cytosine arabinoside in head and neck cancer. *Proc. Am. Assoc. Cancer Res. and ASCO*, 17:248.
7. Jacobs, C. (1980): Cis-platinum versus cis-platinum + methotrexate for the treatment of recurrent head and neck cancer. *Proceedings of the NCI International Head and Neck Oncology Research Conference*, Abstract 2-12.
8. Kaplan, B. H., Schoenfeld, D., and Vogl, S. E. (1981): Treatment of recurrent (Rec) or metastatic (Met) squamous cancer of the head and neck (SCH&N) with methotrexate (M), M plus corynebacterium parvum (CP), or M plus bleomycin (B) plus diamminedichloroplatinum (D). A prospective randomized trial of the Eastern Cooperative Oncology Group. *Proc. Am. Assoc. Cancer Res. and ASCO*, 22:532.
9. Kaplan, B. H., Vogl, S. E., Chiuten, D., Lanham, R., and Wollner, D. (1979): Chemotherapy of advanced cancer of the head and neck with methotrexate, bleomycin, and cis-diamminedichloroplatinum in combination—MBD. *Proc. Am. Assoc. Cancer Res. and ASCO*, 20:384.
10. Kaplan, B. H., Vogl, S. E., and Lerner, H. (1980): Head and neck cancer chemotherapy with diamminodichloroplatinum, bleomycin, methotrexate, and mitomycin MITO-MBD. *Proc. Am. Assoc. Cancer Res. and ASCO*, 21:384.
11. King, G. W., Halpin, J. J., Smith, R. E., Batley, F., and Schuller, D. F. (1979): Cis-diamminedichloroplatinum (II), methotrexate, bleomycin, and vincristine in head and neck cancer: A pilot study. *Cancer Treat. Rep.*, 63:1,735–1,738.
12. Lehane, D. E., Lane, M., Stuckey, W. J., and Dixon, D. (1980): A comparison of methotrexate with methotrexate, methyl CCNU, and bleomycin in patients with advanced squamous cell car-

cinoma of the head and neck region: A Southwest Oncology Group Study. *Proceedings of the NCI International Head and Neck Oncology Research Conference*, Abstract 2-9.

13. Molinari, R., Mattavelli, F., Cantu, G., Chiesa, F., Costa, L., and Tancini, G. (1980): Results of low-dose combination chemotherapy with vincristine, bleomycin, and methotrexate (V-B-M) based on cell kinetics in the palliative treatment of head and neck squamous cell carcinoma. *Eur. J. Cancer*, 16:469–472.

14. Muggia, F. M., Rozencweig, M., and Louie, A. E. (1980): Role of chemotherapy in head and neck cancer: Systemic use of single agents and combinations in advanced disease. *Head Neck Surg.*, 2:196–205.

15. Ratkin, G. A., Brown, C. A., and Ogura, J. H. (1978): Combination chemotherapy in head and neck cancer. *Proc. Am. Assoc. Cancer Res. and ASCO*, 19:330.

16. Wittes, R. E., Spiro, R. H., Shah, J., Gerold, F. P., Koven, B., and Strong, E. W. (1977): Chemotherapy of head and neck cancer: Combination treatment with cyclophosphamide, adriamycin, methotrexate, and bleomycin. *Med. Pediatr. Oncol.*, 3:301–309.

17. Woods, R. L., Stewart, J., Fox, R. M., and Tattersall, M. H. N. (1979): Combination chemotherapy with vincristine, bleomycin, and methotrexate for advanced head and neck cancers. *Cancer Treat. Rep.*, 63:1,997–1,999.

New Approaches in Cancer Therapy,
edited by H. Cortés Funes and M. Rozencweig.
Raven Press, New York © 1982.

The Ingredients of Therapeutic Progress

Franco M. Muggia

*Division of Oncology, Department of Medicine, New York University Medical Center,
New York, New York 10016*

Remarkable progress has been achieved recently in the systemic treatment of breast cancer and germ cell tumors. It is worth commenting on the ingredients of such progress. A similar analysis could be applied to other areas of disease covered in this book; however, it is most striking in these two disease areas.

BREAST CANCER

In breast cancer, the application of adjuvant chemotherapy had resulted in encouraging improvement in survival. A number of second and third generation adjuvant trials have been initiated following the experience from Milano. These are observations extending from the efficacy of chemotherapy, including further intensification of treatment and the addition of endocrine therapies in those groups with the highest rate of relapse.

The determination of estrogen receptors is playing an increasingly large role in the selection of the appropriate hormone alterations and may also have prognostic implications (4). In even earlier stages of disease, trials are being set up first to inquire on the impact of such treatment on survival of patients at lesser risk, and second to seek possible attenuation at local therapies. Additional improvements are likely to be forthcoming through doxorubicin-containing combinations, which are more effective against patients with known metastases (1,2,6). One would anticipate this efficacy to carry over to an even greater extent when given to patients with lesser burdens of disease. As indicated in other parts of the book, new techniques for delivery of doxorubicin and for the monitoring of cardiotoxicity may allow safe testing of such therapies in the adjuvant setting.

Other exciting prospects in the treatment of breast cancer include the introduction of other anthracyclines and new intercalating drugs with possibly improved therapeutic index. Overcoming toxicities, such as alopecia, although mostly a secondary consideration, may also represent an important development for some individuals. Extensive clinical work is ongoing on the integration of these new compounds into our overall clinical strategies. An additional important aspect of research with implications to breast cancer treatment is that concerning the biochemical modulation of 5-fluorouracil. Work on phosphonacetyl-L-aspartate will contribute to our

177

knowledge of the biochemical events of pyrimidine pathways affecting antitumor selectivity. Thus, work on one area of therapeutic research concerning a new agent may contribute towards the efficacy of drugs and drug regimens used in breast cancer chemotherapy. The resulting improvement in our therapeutic approaches is, therefore, related to a matrix of concepts and innovations and not to any one discovery.

GERM CELL TUMORS

In the treatment of germ cell tumors of the testis, the picture is altogether different. Major progress has been achieved by the introduction of a novel cytotoxic drug, cisplatin, into previously modestly effective combination chemotherapeutic regimens (5). In addition, advances in diagnosis, including sensitive biochemical assays for tumor markers and radiographic techniques, have improved our strategies according to stage. The result has been an estimated cure rate exceeding 90%, comprising all stages of the disease, including the most unfavorable histologic types.

The success of cisplatin-containing combinations vindicated the empirical approaches to drug development and the step-wise improvement that occurs through well-designed clinical trials. Germ cell tumors of origins other than the testis are also very responsive to these combinations, as documented by Dr. Cortes Funes' experience.

Therapeutic progress is more difficult to measure in ovarian cancer because of its frequent diffuse intraperitoneal spread and our inability to verify tumor regression by noninvasive diagnostic procedures. Nevertheless, preliminary results at restaging are yielding up to 20% of all patients reverting to a disease-free state with a significant survival advantage over that achieved at comparable stages with alkylating agents (3). In head and neck carcinomas and in lung cancer, regimens leading to a high percentage of tumor regressions are stimulating renewed efforts to treat the vast majority of patients who are deemed incurable. Sporadic evidence of success is appearing even in these previously discouraging areas of research.

The identification of new effective drugs, coupled with concepts and techniques to improve the therapeutic index of established drugs, constitute a most hopeful line of clinical investigation. Clinical trials have been instrumental in the development of these new approaches in cancer therapy. It is therefore important that we continue to encourage the careful recording of clinical experiences, the cross-fertilization of ideas, and the proper climate for their pursuit.

REFERENCES

1. Aisner, J., Weinberg, V., Perloff, M., et al. (1981): Chemoimmunotherapy for advanced breast cancer: A randomized comparison of 6 combinations (CMF, CAF, vs CAFVP) with or without MER immunotherapy. A CALGB study. (Abstract C-433). *Proc. AACR and ASCO*, 21:443.
2. Bull, J. M., Tormey, D. C., Carbone, P. P., Falkson, G., Blom, J., Perlin, E., and Simon, R. (1978): A randomized comparative trial of adriamycin versus methotrexate in combination drug therapy. *Cancer*, 41:1,649–1,657.
3. Holland, J. F., Bruckner, H. W., Cohen, C. J., et al. (1980): Cisplatin therapy of ovarian cancer. In: *Therapeutic Progress in Ovarian Cancer, Testicular Cancer, and the Sarcomas*, edited by

A. T. Van Oosterom, F. M. Muggia, and F. J. Cleton, pp. 41–52. Martinus Nijhoff Publishers, The Hague.
4. Knight, W. A., III, Livingston, R. B., Gregory, E. J., and McGuire, W. L. (1977): Estrogen receptor as an independent prognostic factor for early recurrence in breast cancer. *Cancer Res.*, 37:4,669–4,671.
5. Muggia, F. M., and Jacobs, E. M. (1978): Chemotherapy of testicular cancer: Impact on curability. In: *Advances in Cancer Chemotherapy*, edited by S. R. Carter, A. Goldin, R. Kuretani, G. Mathe, Y. Sakurai, S. Tsukagoshi, and H. Umezawa, pp. 437–452. Japan Science Society Press, Tokyo; University Park Press, Baltimore.
6. Smalley, R. V., Carpenter, J., Bartolucci, A., et al. (1977): A comparison of cyclophosphamide, tine, and prednisone (CMFVP) in patients with metastatic breast cancer. *Cancer*, 40:625–632.

SUBJECT INDEX

Subject Index